Guide to Symptom Relief in Advanced Disease

Fourth Edition

Claud F.B. Regnard
MBChB, BMSC, MRCP

Sue Tempest
RCPh, MSM, MRPharmS, BPharm

Published by Hochland and Hochland Ltd, 174a Ashley Road, Hale, Cheshire, WA15 9SF, England

© Regnard and Tempest, 1998

Fourth edition, second revision

ISBN 1-898507-38-4

British Library Cataloguing in Publication Data
A catalogue record for this book is available from the British Library

Printed by Interprint Ltd, Malta.

To Nina and Paul
for the pleasure they have brought

Contents

CLINICAL DECISIONS

Acknowledgements

We are indebted to our colleagues who kept us on the right track and gave us time and advice. We are grateful to the following colleagues.

Sarah Alport, Ward Manager, St Oswald's Hospice;

Sue Bale, Director of Nursing Research, Wound Healing Research Unit, University of Wales College of Medicine;

Roger Burne, General Practitioner, Helen House Children's Hospice, Oxford;

Mary Comiskey, Consultant in Palliative Medicine, Marie Curie Centre, Newcastle-upon-Tyne;

Ann Faulkner, Professor of Communication in Health Care, University of Sheffield Medical School;

Peter Maguire, Director of Cancer Research Campaign, Psychological Medicine Group, Christie Hospital, Manchester;

Wendy Makin, Consultant in Palliative Care and Oncology, Christie Hospital, Manchester;

Paul MacNamara, Consultant in Palliative Medicine, St Oswald's Hospice;

Kathryn Mannix, Consultant in Palliative Medicine, Marie Curie Centre, Newcastle-upon-Tyne;

Maev O'Rielly, Specialty Registrar in Palliative Medicine, St Oswald's Hospice, Newcastle-upon-Tyne;

Jackie Saunders, Clinical Nurse Specialist, West Suffolk Hospital;

John W. Thompson, Emeritus Professor of Pharmacology, University of Newcastle-upon-Tyne.

We also thank the medical and nursing staff of St Oswald's Hospice, Newcastle-upon-Tyne, who through regular sessions over several months checked through each section for readibility and sense.

Preface

This guide deals with the management of patients with advanced disease. We have strengthened the clinical decision approach based on what the patient has to tell us, and it is our clear intention to use this information from the patient to guide the professional to appropriate management, rather than prescribe a particular approach. We are offering a map for guidance, not a route march!

Once again, this edition has been rewritten and updated to take into account the changes in care that have occurred since 1992. An innovation is that this Guide will be regularly updated on the CLIP (Current Learning in Palliative Care) web site* and all revisions will be in a revised edition produced in the year 2000. Major revisions will still be produced as new editions every five years. As with the previous editions, this new edition has been developed with the advice of a wide cross-section of palliative care professionals.

The most significant change is that the Guide is no longer restricted to cancer and now also includes conditions such as AIDS, motor neurone disease and other life threatening illness. At the request of users we have reinstated sections on drug dosages in children and managing diabetes that were originally in the first and second editions. For the first time there are also sections on psychological problems, including breaking difficult news. Detailed drug information now includes a formulary and is in an updated and expanded section. We have retained the small format so that nurses, doctors and other professional carers can carry it with them and dip into its pages for suggestions. The layout has evolved from the third edition to be easier to read. All management advice is set out in tables, since we expect readers will want to refer frequently to these sections. Readers wishing more detail or information will find this in small type or in the list of references.

The Guide continues to have a strong emphasis on clinical decisions since we believe that these logical series of decisions will simplify the approach to each symptom, making successful management more likely. This leaves the choice of route to the individual patient, partner and professional. We sincerely hope that it will continue to guide professionals in a wide cross-section of caring environments involved in palliating advanced disease.

---

* CLIP (Current Learning in Palliative Care)

Quarterly updates plus access to regularly updated web page
For information
Web page address: www.clip.org.uk
or contact Hochland and Hochland Ltd

Please note

The authors have made every effort to check current datasheets and current literature up to October 1997, but the dosages, indications, contraindications and adverse effects of drugs change over time as new information is obtained. It is the responsibility of the prescriber to check this information with the manufacturer's current drug datasheet and we strongly urge the reader to do this before administering or prescribing any of the drugs in this book.

In addition, palliative care uses a number of drugs for indications or by routes that are not licensed by the manufacturer. In the UK such unlicensed use is allowed, but at the discretion and with the responsibility of the prescriber.

The Consequences of Advanced Disease

Life-threatening, progressing disease is a creeping crisis that invades patients, partners and carers alike. Although some will grow from the experience, it remains a distressing experience for all.

The distress of the patient

Everyday activities become a source of distress and irritation. This requires so much effort that sleep, appetite and concentration are affected, leaving the individual physically and emotionally drained. Activities which once gave life meaning and purpose are curtailed, reduced or abandoned. Suffering, therefore, alters social interactions, reducing an individual's ability or desire to communicate with others, causing that individual to become dissociated from life around them. Valued relationships suffer, as one woman explained:[1]

> "I've come to hate the way I am towards my grandchildren. I love them to bits, I love to see them, but then I just couldn't be bothered with them. I'd get tired easily because of the pain and I didn't have the energy or patience left for them, and I'd be short. I'd never been like that. Their mother stopped bringing them to the house. Now when they visit they treat me like a stranger. It saddens me to think how they will remember me."

The distress of the partners and family

Carers try to be understanding, but often feel 'closed out' by the patient. Used to facing difficulties together, carers find it difficult to reach the patient, producing a feeling of powerlessness. Unprepared for their new role, they learn by trial and error. Not surprisingly, they question their skills and may even question whether they were responsible for the patient's present suffering. They have little time for re-laxation, reflection or for thinking about the future. As the illness progresses, co-ordination of their lives and accepting help becomes more difficult:

> "I used to love the evenings together when the house would be locked up, and we would curl up to watch a film. We can't really do that now, it's difficult to relax, it's always on our mind that they'll be coming to get him ready and put him to bed."[1]

The distress of the professional carers

The sense of isolation in patients and carers is reflected in professionals. They are faced with multiple physical, psychological, spiritual and social issues and yet often have had little or no training in manag-ing these problems. This can cloud judgement so that sensible, caring professionals can produce illogical and inappropriate treatments. The consequence is unrelieved distress. Unrelieved pain persists and sur-veys have shown that severe pain remains unrelieved in over half of cancer patients,[2] and over 60% of AIDS patients.[3,4]

Such distress seems insurmountable. But palliative care is now well established as an effective means of managing such distress. It cannot remove all distress, but provides a path through the distress and confusion that helps the patient, partner, family and professional achieve a worthwhile quality of life.

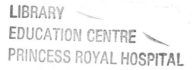

Managing the distress of advanced disease

"I was at home in limbo with this very acute pain. It went on week after week. You begin to give up hope, you think it will never be any better, it would always be there."
*"...the pain was excruciating and I was thinking I can't take any more. I prayed **please** let it be this time."* [1]

Pain and other symptoms often cause psychological distress. Initially, anxiety or a low mood result, and these usually settle rapidly if the symptom is relieved. If, however, the symptom persists or there are fears and unresolved issues around the disease, relationships, beliefs, money or home, the psychological distress will continue and will delay or hamper attempts to manage the symptom. Indeed, it is unusual for a symptom to exist as the only cause of distress, and the phrase 'total pain' was coined by Dame Cicely Saunders to stress the broad nature of such distress in advanced disease. [5]

In such a situation three essential human needs risk becoming blocked: choice (to choose or be chosen), understanding (to understand or be understood), and love (to love or be loved). [6,7] Symptoms such as pain can block choice by limiting actions and plans. Understanding can become blocked if information is not forthcoming or the nature and extent of the symptom is not believed. Love can become blocked by the effect of anger, irritability or low mood on close relationships. The result of blocking choice are frustration, anger and bitterness, blocking understanding causes fear and anxiety, while blocking love causes isolation and loneliness. If any of the feelings persist, depression is often the result. Sometimes patients develop behaviours which further complicate treatment and recovery:

Issues around these needs must be addressed. [8] The support and co-operation of the interprofessional team (nurses, doctors, specialists, social worker, physiotherapist, occupational therapist, pharmacist and others) is necessary to achieve success. Help starts with assessment and supportive communication. Anxiety, anger and depression in particular need to managed. The full range of additional treatments possible is wide and depends on the enthusiasm of the team, but includes touch, [9] hypnosis, [10,11] art therapy, [12] music therapy, [13] imagery, [14] and aromatherapy. When the psychological distress is severe, expert help will be required. The skills needed may be those of cognitive therapy, psychiatry, or family therapy, although the choice sometimes depends on availability of personnel rather than suitability of the approach.

An intelligent young woman developed recurrence of breast cancer. For several months she had suffered severe chest pain. On admission to a palliative care unit the pain failed to respond to several strong opioids or to a range of secondary analgesics, including ketamine. Spinal analgesia relieved her pain but only partially relieved her distress. Despite a change of antidepressant suggested by the psychiatrist, she remained severely depressed and she became increasingly demanding of extra analgesia, culminating in throwing herself out of bed or chair, and screaming out her demands for sedation. Distraction, relaxation, aromatherapy were minimally helpful, whilst imagery gave some insights into her distress, but no relief. It became increasingly difficult to care for her. With advice and help the professional team began a behavioural programme, negotiating increasingly longer times without demands, and rewarding success with attention and time. Gradually the behaviour resolved sufficiently to allow her to be admitted for the neurosurgical procedure of rhizotomy, with complete resolution of her pain

Principles of Symptom Management

- **Effective palliative care is the right of every patient and partner, and the duty of every professional.**
Access to training, updating, and to specialist palliative care services should be widely available.
- **Ensure adequate team skills, knowledge, attitudes and communication.**
Individuals and teams need basic skills in communication and diagnosis, together with the knowledge of symptoms in advanced disease, their effects and management.
- **Create a safe place to suffer .**
This is not a building, but the relationship between carer and patient, one that enables the patient to feel safe to express their distress. Not all distress can be removed, but the expression of that distress is therapeutic.[15]
- **Establish a partnership with the patient, the partner and family.**
The flow of information and treatment decisions should be controlled by the patient and negotiated with the partner and family.
- **Do not wait for a patient to complain — ask and observe.**
Patients with persistent distress do not always look distressed. They may be withdrawn, with poor sleep or mobility, and the effects of the pain may have spilt over into the partner or relative. Assessing these factors is more important than estimating severity which open to bias and often unhelpful in deciding treatment. The comments of the partner or relative are often helpful.
- **Accurately diagnose the cause of the problem.**
Problems are often multiple and mixed. In advanced cancer, for example, 85% of patients have more than one site of pain, and 40% have four or more pains.[16]
- **Clinical estimates of symptom severity are highly subjective and are a poor basis for choosing a treatment.**
A successful choice requires a clear diagnosis together with the willingness to modify the choice depending on the response. This tailors the treatment to the patient.
- **Do not delay starting treatment.**
Symptoms should be treated promptly since they become more difficult to treat the longer they are left. This is partly because their persistence makes it increasingly difficult for the patient to cope. In neuropathic pain, for example, the longer pain the persists, the more pathways and receptors are involved, making control much more difficult. Treatment must start as soon as the diagnosis is made.
- **Administer drugs regularly in doses titrated to each individual, that ensure the symptom does not return.**
If a drug gives effective relief for 4 hours, then prescribe it 4-hourly. 'As required' or 'PRN' administration on its own will not control continuous symptoms.
- **Set realistic goals.**
Firstly accept the patient's goals. If these seem overly optimistic, negotiate some additional *shorter* term goals. If the patient's goals seem overly pessimistic then negotiate some additional *longer* term goals. A clear plan of action based on negotiated goals helps the patient and partner see a way out of their distress.
- **Re-assess repeatedly and regularly.**
Accurate titration of medication demands reassessment.
- **Treat concurrent symptoms.**
Patients with other symptoms such as nausea and breathlessness experience more pain than those without these symptoms.[17]
- **Empathy, understanding, diversion and elevation of mood are essential adjuncts.**
Drugs are only part of overall management.

Setting the scene for an interview

Clinical decision	If YES → Action

• Greet person and introduce yourself by name and position

IS THE PERSON ACCOMPANIED?	• Ask if it is possible to see the person on their own *If person agrees:* arrange to see them alone. *If person disagrees:* see them with accompanying person and arrange to see person alone at a later interview.
IS TIME SHORT?	**If less than 30 minutes available or patient too unwell for full interview:** • Focus on recent changes or major problems only

• Explain your role and objectives

DOES THE PERSON OBJECT TO THESE?	• Explore the reasons: *If the person refuses further negotiation:* offer help if needed. No further action. *If person agrees:* renegotiate objectives, eg. concentrate on main problem only.

• Mention the time available

DOES PERSON OBJECT TO TIME AVAILABLE?	**If time is too short:** • Explore the reasons and try to negotiate follow up interviews. *If person objects to negotiation:* acknowledge this and end interview. *If person agrees to negotiation:* arrange longer interview for later. **If time is too long:** Explore reasons and negotiate more limited objectives eg. main problem only.

• Mention that you would like to take notes during the interview

DOES PERSON OBJECT TO YOU TAKING NOTES?	• Explore the reasons: *If person objects to negotiation:* agree not to take notes. *If person agrees to negotiation:* take notes of what has been agreed (person may ask for some information to be left unrecorded).

• Mention that you are part of a team and need to share what is discussed with colleagues.

DOES THE PERSON OBJECT TO SHARING INFORMATION WITH TEAM?	eg. person insists that some or all information is kept secret • Advise person that you cannot agree to secrecy *If person objects:* offer to refer to a professionally supported counsellor. *If person agrees:* go on to elicit the current problems.

Adapted from Maguire, Faulkner and Regnard [18]

NOTES

Seeing the person alone will result in more disclosure of the person's concerns.[18] This needs to be balanced against the important need to include partners and relatives in the care. It is common practice in palliative care, therefore, to see patients and partners together on the first interview, and then to see individuals on their own at later stage. **Time available for interview:** at least 30 minutes is needed to elicit the persons problems, and they dislose them more quickly if they know how much time is available. **Taking notes and sharing information:** it is essential to make notes of important cues and issues because it shows the person you are taking their problems seriously. It does not hinder disclosure and gives you a record for the future. Sharing information is essential to team working and makes best use of the team's pooled expertise. It also reduces the risk of dependency on the professional, unrealistic expectations and over-dependency.[18]

Eliciting the current problems

Clinical decision	If YES → Action

- Ask about current problems
- Avoid interruption
- Summarise problems
- Screen again (eg. Before I talk to you about these problems, are there any other problems?)

IS THERE AN OVER-RIDING PRIORITY?	• Explain priority (eg. 'We need to deal with this pain first'). • See appropriate clinical decision table for guidance to management. • Return later to complete interview.
IS PERSON UNABLE TO PRIORITISE?	• Focus on the first problem chosen or mentioned.

- Identify each problem in turn
- Clarify the precise nature of the problem
- Specify severity and duration

IS PROBLEM CAUSING ANY DISTRESS?	eg. 'How have you been feeling about this?' **If person is obviously distressed:** • Acknowledge distress. • *If person can bear to talk about it:* identify, clarify and specify each emotion. • *If person cannot bear to talk about it:* agree to leave this problem.
IS TIME FOR INTERVIEW ENDING?	• Explain that time is nearly up. • Summarise issues • Check if there is anything the person wants to add. • Make concluding statement. • Arrange next interview.

Adapted from Maguire, Faulkner and Regnard [18]

NOTES

Eliciting problems: this is easier if the person can describe problems in their own way without interruption. Summarising demonstrates you were listening and makes sure the problem list is correct.

Identify each problem in turn, making sure both of you are talking about the same problem.

Clarify the precise nature of the problem, what it is like, what effects it has.

Specify the duration of the problem, whether it is continuous or intermittent, when it started and its severity.

Distress: disclosure of emotions is more likely to happen if feelings have been mentioned in the first 10 minutes of an interview.[19] Patients or partners who are distressed would like this acknowledged, together with help to understand why they are feeling this way. Professionals often feel anxious when this distress is openly expressed, fearing that they have 'upset' the person or caused psychological damage. Harm will only occur if the professional insists on talking about a problem they the individual has stated is too difficult to discuss.

Concluding the interview: this is as important as starting the interview. If the professional does not finish within the agreed time the person may think they have unlimited time and demand more time which prevents the professional spending time with other patients.

Breaking difficult news

Clinical decision	If YES → Action

- Difficult news cannot be made easier, but telling it badly creates new difficulties.
- It is the patient who decides how much should be told.
- Denial helps patients to cope.
- Collusion is usually an act of caring

IS THE PERSON UNABLE TO UNDERSTAND?	• *If this is reversible* (eg. deafness responding to a hearing aid): treat the cause. • *If this is irreversible:* unless patient has previously objected, inform relative or partner of the difficult news, using these clinical decisions.
IS RELATIVE OR PARTNER COLLUDING?	ie. wanting to withhold information from patient. • Accept that carer does know patient better than any professional. • Explore reasons for collusion (remember that the carer is doing what they think best at the time) • Ask for permission to find out from patient what they are think of the situation. • Check the cost of collusion on the patient-carer relationship.
IS THE SETTING INAPPROPRIATE?	• Find somewhere confidential and, if possible, quiet, comfortable and free from interruptions. • Ask if the person would like someone else to be present.

- **Ask what the person already knows** (eg. Can you tell me what you understand is happening?)
- **Check their understanding** (eg. What do you make of what s happening?)

DOES THE PERSON ALREADY KNOW?	**If the person does not need more information:** • *For the patient:* go to decisions on helping with the effects of difficult news. • *For partner or relative:* if patient agrees, inform person of the patient's level of knowledge. **If more information is requested:** • *If the additional information is difficult news:* give 'warning shot' as below. • *If the additional information is **not** difficult news:* supply the information (ideally with written or taped backup) and go to decisions on helping with the effects of bad news.

- **Warn:** give warning shot (eg. The test results are more serious than we thought.).
- **Pause** to allow person to respond.
- **Check** if the person wants to continue (eg. Do you want me to explain further?).

HAS PERSON RESPONDED TO THE 'WARNING SHOT'?	eg. 'What do you mean, more serious?' or 'Are you saying it's cancer?' • Continue with Warn, Pause, Check -answer invitation for more information (eg. 'We found some abnormal cells'). -ensure person understands this information. -keep giving information as long as person continues to request information

Adapted from Faulkner, Maguire, Regnard [20]

NOTES

Difficult news: this any news that is unexpected and may cause distress. It is usually 'bad' news, but this label is one decided by care professionals. There are occasions when apparently 'good' news causes as much distress as 'bad' news. For example, the news that radiotherapy for a frontal lobe brain tumour has resulted in a long remission may seem good news from a professional's view, but could be devastating to a relative who has now to cope with months or years of someone with an altered personality.

Setting and information: two essential preparatory stages are ensuring an appropriate environment (a busy corridor is unacceptable), and asking what the person already knows. It is often helpful for the person to have a friend, partner or another professional for support and to clarify issues.

Warn, Pause, Check: these simple three steps ensure the person can have information given at their pace and at a level and amount they can cope with. Some persons will push the process along quickly (eg. 'So it's cancer, I thought so.'), while others will slow up the process (eg. 'I'm not sure I want to go into the details now.').

Helping with the effects of difficult news

Clinical decision	If YES → Action

- **Pause** to check the person s reaction.
- **Acknowledge** any distress.

IS THE PERSON ACCEPTING THE DIFFICULT NEWS?	• Acknowledge and explore any feelings and concerns. • Monitor regularly for feelings of defeat, spiritual anguish, anger and withdrawal (see **the Angry person**, and **the Withdrawn patient**).
IS THE PERSON OVERWHELMINGLY DISTRESSED?	• Acknowledge the distress. • Explore the individual concerns to work out why the reaction has been so disturbing.
IS THE PERSON DENYING OR HOLDING ON TO UNREALISTIC EXPECTATIONS?	• **If the person is coping well with these feelings:** Do not persist in challenging denial or unrealistic expectations (after all, they **are** coping!). **If the person is not coping with these feelings:** • Acknowledge denial or unrealistic expectations. • Check for a window on the denial (eg. 'Are there times, even for a second, when you're less sure that everything is all right?'). • Gently challenge inconsistencies (eg. 'You say everything is fine, but you're still losing in weight.') • Avoid being defensive about unrealistic expectations
IS THE PERSON AMBIVALENT?	• Acknowledge the uncertainty (eg. 'It seems that you're uncertain.') • Offer time for help (eg. 'When you need more information, just ask.').
IS THE PATIENT COLLUDING?	• Recognise that this is often due to a need to protect the partner. • Accept that the patient does know the partner or relative better than any professional. • Explore the reasons for the collusion and check the cost of that collusion. • Ask for permission to speak to the partner or relative to find out what they think about the situation.

Adapted from Faulkner, Maguire, Regnard[20]

NOTES

The effects of difficult news: faced with difficult news most people respond with acceptance or denial. Some will be firm in this reaction while many will fluctuate between the two, sometimes during one conversation (one young woman with weeks to live said to us, 'I know I'm going to die soon, but I've booked my holiday next year anyway.'). A few people will be half way in between, ambivalent about whether they want to know more.

Overwhelming distress: mixed with these reactions will be a wide range of possible reactions such as anger, bitterness, sadness, and fear. Sometimes this is expressed openly at the time of understanding the difficult news. Professionals are often fearful of this reaction and worry that they have 'upset' the person or caused psychological damage. As long as the disclosure has been at the person's pace with them in control, no damage will be caused. Open expression can be helpful to the individual and allows the professional to explore feelings further.

Coping with denial or unrealistic expectations: there is often a perception that these reactions are abnormal and will harm or delay the person's 'acceptance' of the situation. In reality, these reactions are important and powerful protective mechanisms for anyone facing difficult news. They key is not whether they exist, but whether their presence is working to help the individual cope. If the person is coping then no action need be and thoughtless intervention shows little regard for the patient, partner and family.[21] Obviously if these reactions are failing to protect the individual, then gently challenging the presence of denial or unrealistic expectations may enable the person to express their distress more clearly. This expression is in itself therapeutic and may lead to some resolution of that distress.

Collusion: this can be with the patient, the partner, or both. Collusion is another reaction that is seen as abnormal by professionals. Collusion by an individual is often an act of love, protecting someone they love and know well. This reaction is understandable and like denial can be left if it is working for those involved. Collusion can cause difficulties if it is damaging the relationship through a 'conspiracy of silence', in which case this cost will need to be explored and gently challenged.

Handling difficult questions

Clinical decision	If YES → Action

- **Acknowledge the importance of the question**
- **Offer a quieter location if the first is awkward.**
- **Check why the question is being asked** (eg. I wonder why you re asking me this now?)

IS PERSON RELUCTANT TO PURSUE QUESTION?	**If they misunderstood your question:** • Check for deafness, drowsiness or confusion. • Ask in a different way. **If you were unprepared for question (or unwilling to listen):** • Apologise for the inattention. • Show that you **are** listening by repeating the person's question. • Acknowledge again its importance. • Negotiate if they wish to continue or speak to someone else. **If you are uncomfortable with the question:** • Don't be afraid to describe your feelings (eg. 'I'm finding that difficult to answer.' or 'I don't know what to say.') **If the person is clear about wanting to stop the interview:** • Acknowledge the refusal. Let the person know they are free to ask again in the future.
IS A CLEAR ANSWER DIFFICULT?	ie. your response will face the person with uncertainty (eg. possible response: 'I don't know how much time is left.'). • Acknowledge uncertainty and the pain it causes (eg. 'I can see this uncertainty is difficult for you.') • Explore if person can accept small chunks of certainty such as understanding what is known of the illness (eg. 'How does it look to you at the moment?'). • If person needs to make realistic plans, give a 'best guess' response making clear that this is based on experience, not certainty.
IS THE ANSWER DIFFICULT NEWS?	• Follow the clinical decisions in **Breaking difficult news**.
IS A CLEAR ANSWER POSSIBLE?	• Provide answer or information.

Adapted from Faulkner and Regnard [22]

NOTES

Difficult questions: many factors can make some questions difficult.[22,23] *For the patient and partner* there is a need for information to make rational choices, but this may conflict with the fears of advancing illness (treatment, symptoms, emotions, dying, relationships and finances) and the need to maintain hope in the face of uncertainty. These factors inevitably generate difficult questions. *For the professional* there are fears of being blamed, of eliciting a emotional reaction, of admitting ignorance, of expressing emotions, of medical hierarchy and of doing something for which they have received little or no training.[23] These factors make the questions of a patient or partner more difficult to answer.

Approaching difficult questions: although the setting has been chosen by the questioner this may have been opportunistic and it is reasonable to offer a quieter location if the original location is awkward such as a busy corridor. It is important to acknowledge the thought, anxiety and courage it may have taken to ask the question. Checking why the question is being asked avoids misunderstandings (one doctor was asked, 'How much longer?' only to find the patient wanted to know if the appointment would finish in time for lunch!). Some questioners will be reluctant to pursue the question, but the reasons for this need to be understood. If the professional feels uncomfortable with the question it is helpful to admit this both to themselves and to the questioner. Often the answer has to be vague because certainty is lacking, but it is important to make this clear. If the answer is likely to be difficult news then using the clinical decisions in **Breaking difficult news** allows the questioner to take the information at their pace.

Introduction: **NOTES AND REVISIONS** (regular revision updates available on CLIP update service)

Clinical
Decisions
in
Symptom
Management

"You believe there is nothing more that can be done, that's it, you are completely on your own."

A patient [1]

- Work through these 10 clinical decisions in order – these cover most pains seen in advanced disease.
- Use the information provided to help you decide which pain is present.
- Follow the suggestions for managing the pain- use the notes for more information.
- For details on using analgesics, see Drug Formulary section.

Clinical decision	If YES → Action
1 **IS THE PAIN SEVERE AND OVERWHELMING?**	**Immediate:** achieve sufficient comfort to allow initial assessment. • *For severe pain related to the slightest passive movement:* find comfortable position (padding/splint). Give diamorphine SC, IM or IV (5mg if not on opioid, otherwise use equivalent of usual 4-hourly dose). • *For agitation that prevents assessment:* give midazolam 5mg SC **or** titrate 1-5mg IV • *For colic:* hyoscine butylbromide 20mg SC, IM or IV *Choice of route:* SC is kindest but slowest, use IM or IV if rapid response needed.(minimum wait for reassessment after SC = 30mins; after IM = 20mins; after IV= 2mins) **Within 1 hour:** exclude causes requiring urgent management. • *For back pain:* exclude cord compression- see Emergencies (Cord compression) • *If pathological fracture suspected:* decide if patient is able to travel for X-ray. • *For a myocardial infarction:* treat as appropriate. **Within 4 hours:** achieve comfort at rest • *If still in pain at rest:* if not on an opioid, start morphine. Otherwise increase regular opioid dose by 50%. Consider contacting pain or palliative care specialist. • *If several opioid dose increases have been ineffective:* try ketamine (see **Drug formulary** for details). • *If still in pain at rest and further treatment is to be delayed for more than 6 hours:* consider light sedation with SC infusion of midazolam 30mg per 24 hours plus diamorphine at equivalent of current dose (see p19 for equivalent doses). **Within 24 hours:** plan for stable pain control. • Check through the following Clinical decisions 2-10. • Ensure a good night's sleep using sedatives if necessary. • If the pain is localised (eg. fracture), consider spinal analgesia or a nerve block. **Within 1 week:** plan for managing any psychological consequences • See sections on **Anxiety**, **Anger**, **Withdrawal** (the presence of these problems may delay resolution of the pain for several weeks).

Adapted from Thompson and Regnard [4]

Notes

1 Severe or overwhelming pain

Severe pain causes considerable distress, and needs to be treated promptly. The aim is to tackle each stage within the time suggested, while planning the next step. the most immediate goal is to reduce pain at rest and to allow the patient to settle sufficiently to allow adequate assessment.

Overwhelming pain: distress can make it more difficult to cope with any pain. If both increase and remain untreated the distress and pain can merge to create a situation which overwhelms the patient. This can happen within hours and prevents the patient from clearly expressing their problem- they may even say that the pain is 'all over' their body. If this is accompanied by agitation, treatment needs to be prompt. Some patients will require no more than 2.5mg midazolam IM (eg. ill patients or those who have slept little in the previous 24 hours), others will require more than 10mg (eg. younger patients or those previously on benzodiazepines). Although the agitation may settle, low mood, anxiety and exhaustion may persist (see sections on **Anxiety**, **Anger**, **Withdrawal**). This persistence of psychological problems will delay the resolution of the pain for several weeks and to avoid disappointment this needs to be understood by patient, partner and staff.[2]

Clinical decision	If YES → Action
2 **IS THE PAIN RELATED TO MOVEMENT?** **(ie. worsened or precipitated by movement)**	**a) Worsened by the slightest passive movement** • *Fracture* (deformity may be present): immobilise /see clinical decision 1 for severe pain. Consider elective orthopaedic surgery and radiotherapy if due to a metastasis. • *Severe soft tissue inflammation:* usually due to infection: see red/ hot skin (Clinical decision 7). If infection is deeper, movement pain may be the only sign. • *Inflammation or irritation of muscle* (affected muscle in spasm): see 2c below. • *Nerve compression:* see Clinical decision 9. **b) Worsened by straining bone during examination** (eg. percussing spine, pressing rib) • Consider nerve compression (see Clinical decision 9) or bone infection (see notes). • *Bone metastases* (may need to be confirmed on bone scan): If in pain at rest, start a strong opioid and increase by 50% every 3rd day if needed. If no improvement after several dose increases, add a NSAID for one week's trial (eg. diclofenac or ibuprofen). For single site pain arrange radiotherapy. If pain is in multiple sites use a pamidronate infusion 60-90mg repeated every 1-3 months. Consider referral for Strontium [3] or hemibody irradiation. **c) Worsened by active movement** (ie. movement against resistance) • *Skeletal instability:* pain on minimal active movement such as coughing or standing suggests there is a risk of bone fracture or collapse. Treat bone metastases as in Clinical decision 2b above. Arrange for an urgent X-ray and consider referral for orthopaedic and radiotherapy opinion. • *Myofascial pain* (myotomal distribution, trigger point (TP) in muscle which reproduces pain when pressed): inject TP with 0.25% bupivacaine or use TENS over TP. • *Skeletal muscle strain* (history of sudden onset during exertion): TENS, local cold.

Clinical decision	If YES → Action
2 (cont) **IS THE PAIN RELATED TO MOVEMENT?** **(ie. worsened or precipitated by movement)**	**d) Worsened by inspiration** • *Rib metastases* (local tenderness is present): intercostal nerve block (bupivacaine 0.25% and 40mg methylprednisolone), for multiple sites see Clinical decision 2b). • *Pleuritic pain* (local rub may be present): consider an embolus (treatment not usually necessary). Treat infection if present. Consider a NSAID + intercostal block. • *Peritoneal pain due to local inflammation* (eg. metastasis involving peritoneum):NSAID (eg. diclofenac or ibuprofen). If the pain is localised to one or two dermatomes, try an intercostal block. **e) Consider also:** • *Arthritis (inflammatory or infective):* treat local infection if this is present / start NSAID (eg. diclofenac or ibuprofen). • *Gastric distension due to gastric stasis* (fullness, early satiation, hiccups, heartburn): metoclopramide or domperidone. Consider cisapride. • *Local distension due to haemorrhage:* exclude bleeding disorder. Consider opioid or ketamine (see **Drug formulary**). • *Local distension due to tumour:* Strong opioid + high dose dexamethasone. A local block or spinal analgesia is sometimes needed. • *Local inflammation due to tumour, infection or trauma:* exclude and treat infection. Try topical or systemic NSAID. Consider topical morphine[10, 11] or radiotherapy if this is tumour.

Adapted from Thompson and Regnard [4]

Notes

2: Pain related to movement

Fracture: movement of the affected part by the examiner will usually result in severe pain on the slightest movement. Pathological fractures (eg. bone metastases) are not always painful when they occur, but pain is usually a feature within minutes. Follow the advice for severe pain in clinical decision 1.

Bone metastases or infection: local tenderness over a bone suggests a local weakness. In immunocompromised patients infection should be excluded, especially mycobacteria. Bone metastases are best picked up on bone scan, except for myeloma and renal carcinoma which may show better up on X-rays. If severe enough, skeletal instability can cause pain on minimal active movement such as coughing. The aim is to stabilise the unstable skeleton. Initially this is done by immobilisation and external splinting. The primary cause of the instability then needs to be treated (eg. radiotherapy for bone metastases). Occasionally, operative fixation is necessary. The pain of multiple metastases require systemic treatments, the simplest of which is an intravenous infusion of bisphosphonates such as pamidronate or clodronate,[5, 6] Strontium-89 is an effective, but more expensive and complicated alternative.[3] When used regularly bisphosphonates have the added advantage of reducing skeletal complications.[7, 8]

Myofascial pain: this pain is common in advanced disease and should always be looked for in movement related pains. The pain is distributed in a myotomal pattern. Charts showing the typical distribution of all the main muscles are available.[9] A trigger point is usually present in the affected muscle and consists of a single spot which produces the pain when pressed with band of muscle in spasm palpable beneath the trigger point..

Skeletal muscle strain: this occurs suddenly during exertion. Local warmth is more pleasant to apply, but local cold is effective for longer.

Inflammation or irritation of muscle: infection or tumour involving muscle will cause that muscle to go into painful spasm. Involvement of the psoas muscle, for example, causes painful hip flexion on that side. Infection must be excluded and treated if present. The pain of tumour infiltration can be helped with dexamethasone + a local nerve or spinal block.

Severe soft tissue inflammation: this is usually due to an acute infection. Overlying skin is usually red and swollen, and antibiotics are indicated (see Clinical decision 7). Deeper infections or those in AIDS patients may have few signs. In head and neck cancer, the rapid onset of severe pain may be the only symptom: treatment with a combination of flucloxacillin and metronidazole will quickly ease the pain. In patients with AIDS a deeper infection may be an abscess which needs draining and IV antibiotics.

Pleuritic pain: this is due to local inflammation and persistent pain can be eased with a NSAID or an intercostal block of the affected area.

Other causes: structures that are inflamed, infected or distended may cause pain on movement.

Clinical decision	If YES → Action
3 **IS THE PAIN PERIODIC?** (ie. comes and goes regularly every few minutes)	**Abdominal pain** • *Constipation, bowel obstruction, or bowel irritation* (drugs, radiotherapy, chemotherapy, infection). Treat cause, but for relief use hyoscine butylbromide 10-20mg SC as required. Can be used as continuous SC infusion (30-180mg per 24 hrs). **Suprapubic pain with urinary frequency or urgency** • *Bladder colic due to:* infection, outflow obstruction, unstable bladder, irritation by tumour. Treat cause, but for relief use hyoscine butylbromide as above. See **Urinary problems.** **Loin pain radiating to groin** • *Ureteric colic due to infection or obstruction.* Treat cause, but for relief use diclofenac 75mg IM or 100mg PR. Consider hyoscine butylbromide as above.
4 **IS THE PAIN RELATED TO A PROCEDURE?**	eg. dressing change. • Change the technique (eg. different dressings or using the topical anaesthetic EMLA) • Try Entonox (50% nitrous oxide, 50% oxygen) **if** available **and** patient can comply. • Try a 4-hourly dose of usual analgesic given PO or SC(see p19 for equivalents). • Consider:Sedation with midazolam 1-5mg titrated IV **or** 2.5-5mg SC. Ketamine (see **Drug formulary** for details).
5 **IS THE PAIN RELATED TO EATING?**	**Pain in the mouth** See **Oral problems.** **Pain on swallowing** See **Dysphagia.** **Abdominal pain** • *Gastritis:* treat cause. Consider ranitidine. If bleeding is present add sucralfate suspension 10mls 6 hourly as a haemostatic agent. • *Duodenitis:* ranitidine. • *Gastric stasis causing heartburn:* metoclopramide or domperidone. Consider cisapride.

Adapted from Thompson and Regnard[4]

Notes

3 Periodic pain (colic)

Smooth muscle spasm causes regular episodes of pain lasting a few minutes. This periodic feature is characteristic of colic, although occasionally, colic is continuous. Bowel is the commonest source, followed by bladder and ureter. Bile duct is an unusual source. Opioids are ineffective and may worsen the pain. A smooth muscle relaxant (antispasmodic) is the treatment of choice. Hyoscine butylbromide (Buscopan) is preferred since it has fewer central effects than hyoscine hydrobromide.

4 Pain related to a procedure

Procedures that are painful produce increasing fear and pain with future procedures. Adequate analgesia or sedation prevent this build up of anxiety.

5 Pain related to eating

Pain will be caused by anything which causes inflammation of the mucosa of the mouth, pharynx, oesophagus or stomach. Related structures must also be considered such as teeth. See **Oral problems** and **Dysphagia.**

Clinical decision	If YES → Action
6 **IS THE PAIN MADE WORSE BY PASSING URINE OR STOOL?**	**Pain on micturition** • See **Urinary problems**. **Pain on passing stool** • Consider: hard stool (see **Constipation**), haemorrhoids (use topical soothing cream), infection (treat), local tumour (see 2e), tenesmoid pain (see Clinical decision 8).
7 **ARE THERE ASSOCIATED SKIN CHANGES?**	• *Pressure sore:* benzydamine cream or ibuprofen gel to ulcer edge 8-12 hourly. See **Skin pressure damage** • *Malignant ulcer:* See **Malignant ulcers** • *Red /hot skin:* Exclude eczema or dermatitis. If cellulitis is suspected start antibiotic (penicillin V or erythromycin in lymphoedematous limb, otherwise use flucloxacillin). Consider if this pain may be a sympathetic hypoactivity pain (see Clinical decision 8). • *Pale/cold skin:* if this is arterial insufficiency contact a vascular surgeon for advice. An opioid is only partly effective, and alternatives are ketamine (see **Drug formulary** for details), or a local nerve or spinal block. Also consider if this pain is a sympathetic hyperactivity pain (see Clinical decision 8). • *For other skin disease:* treat the cause.
8 **ARE THERE UNPLEASANT SENSORY CHANGES AT REST?**	Neuropathic pain is a general term describing pain in which patients describe altered sensation (reduced, sensitive or painful to touch), and describe unusual unpleasant sensations such as burning, stinging, stabbing. There are three types of neuropathic pain: **Pain in a dermatome** (ie. in the distribution of a spinal nerve root eg.L1) =deafferentation pain: • Start low dose amitriptyline (10-25mg once at night) and titrate. If adverse effects are troublesome, try imipramine (10-25mg at night and titrate). If the pain is no better, add sodium valproate 200mg 12 - hourly and titrate. Advice from a pain or palliative care specialist is usually needed if the pain persists, and possibilities include using ketamine, nerve blocks or spinal drugs. **Pain in area supplied by peripheral nerve** =neuropathy or neuralgia: • Exclude reversible causes (eg. B12 deficiency). Treat as for deafferentation pain. **Pain in a sympathetic distribution** (ie. the same distribution as the arterial supply since sympathetic nerves run along arteries) = sympathetically maintained pain: • Start treating in the same way as deafferentation pain. If the skin is cold and pale, this is hyperactive sympathetic activity and a pain specialist may advise a chemical sympathectomy. If skin is warm and red or dusky, this is hypoactive sympathetic activity and this can sometimes be helped by placing TENS electrodes over the main artery supplying the area (do not use this over the carotids in the neck).

Clinical decision	If YES → Action
9 **IS THE PAIN IN AN AREA SUPPLIED BY A NERVE?**	• If this is an unpleasant sensory change at rest: see Clinical decision 8. • *Nerve compression:* Start an opioid. Exclude whether the nerve compression is being caused by skeletal instability with X-rays ± bone scan (a CAT or MRI scan may be necessary). Exclude or treat bone infection. For tumours or metastases consider dexamethasone (16mg daily reducing to 4-6mg) or radiotherapy. A TENS may help. Occasionally a nerve block or spinal analgesia is needed.
10 **IS THE PAIN PERSISTING?**	• Consider -unresolved fear, anger or depression (see **Anxiety**, **Anger**, **Withdrawal**). -poor compliance because of fear, misunderstanding of instructions or an unacceptable form of medication. -inappropriate analgesic dose or timing. -onset of a new pain (go through previous 9 Clinical decisions).

Adapted from Thompson and Regnard [4]

Notes

6 Pain worsened by passing urine or stool

Problems such as urinary infection or constipation can cause pain.

7 Associated skin changes

Ulcers: the most painful part of an ulcer is usually the damaged skin edge. Application of a NSAID cream or gel can be effective.[12] When pain is due to damage to deeper structures, opioids or local nerve or spinal block may be needed. See **Skin pressure damage** and **Malignant ulcers**.

8 Unpleasant sensory changes at rest

Neuropathic pain is due to persistent changes in the spinal cord in receptor and neurotransmitter functioning.[13] The term covers deafferentation pain (due to altered sensory processing following previous nerve damage causing pain in a dermatomal distribution), sympathetically maintained pain (pain in an autonomic nerve distribution), painful peripheral neuropathies, and peripheral neuralgias. Treatment can be complex,[14] and the advice of a pain specialist can be invaluable. Opioids may be helpful, but secondary analgesics (eg. tricyclic antidepressants) can be effective.

9 Nerve compression

If the cause is a tumour the aim is to shrink the tumour (eg. radiotherapy) or reduce the oedema around the tumour with dexamethasone. A local nerve or spinal block may be needed.

10 Persistent pain

If pain persists despite going through these clinical decisions, then a complete reassessment is necessary. A new pain or poor compliance are common reasons for persistent pain. It is also important to exclude unresolved psychological issues, since these reduce the ability to cope with pain and may produce pain behaviours. These will need to be addressed.

Using Opioids

The modified analgesic ladder for opioid responsive pain

If no analgesic: Start paracetamol PO 0.5 - 1G 4-hourly.
  If already on paracetamol: change to low dose morphine (eg. 10-30mg daily).
    If patient finds change to morphine unacceptable, then change to a weak opioid.
      If already on weak opioid: change to morphine (eg. 30-60mg daily)
        or equivalent strong opioid agonist.
          If already on morphine: consider intraspinal morphine or look for alternative
            approaches (eg. secondary analgesics, nerve blocks, radiotherapy).

This stepped approach only applies to choosing an analgesic for opioid responsive pain. The original ladder includes a weak opioid as a middle step.[15] Weak opioids are a useful step if strong opioids are difficult to obtain, or patients are too fearful of strong opioids. If a patient is on a weak opioid, and pain is still present, there is no advantage to switching to a different weak opioid. If strong opioids are easily available then it is possible to miss the middle step altogether by moving from a nonopioid to a low dose of a strong opioid.

Strong opioids

Morphine is the strong opioid of choice, with extensive experience and research demonstrating its value in the pains of advanced disease. The mouth is the route of choice (as an instant release tablet or solution, or controlled release tablets, capsules or suspension), but alternatives are the rectal, subcutaneous and spinal routes.

Diamorphine is useful subcutaneously, since its high solubility allows for lower volumes of administration.

Hydromorphone may be the preferred alternative to morphine since it does not appear to have the complex pharmacokinetics of methadone or transdermal fentanyl. It is useful when morphine is not tolerated because of adverse effects or in the presence of renal impairment.

Transdermal fentanyl is a useful alternative when a non-oral route is required. It can also be used in renal impairment, but there are delays in reaching a steady plasma level on starting, and longer delays on blood levels returning to normal after stopping the drug.

Methadone can be used in the presence of renal impairment and has NMDA antagonist activity. It accumulates and requires careful titration (see **Drug formulary**).

Other opioids have no advantages over these strong opioids.

Which dose?

- **Opioid requirements depend on previous analgesic needs, renal function and age.**
- **Recommended 'maximum' doses have no relevance to the control of pain in advanced disease.**

Weight, height and surface area correlate poorly with the amount of opioid needed. Morphine is absorbed from the small bowel, metabolised in the liver to an active and potent analgesic metabolite (morphine-6-glucuronide, M6G) which is then excreted through the kidney.[16, 17] Although hepatic dysfunction has some effect on morphine metabolism,[18] it requires severe hepatic failure to have a clinical impact, and such levels of failure are rare in advanced disease. In contrast, any reduction in renal function will result in the accumulation of M6G and a second metabolite, M3G with resulting adverse effects.[19, 20] This is not usually a problem if the morphine dose is reduced to take the impaired renal function into account. The effects of hydromorphone, fentanyl and methadone are not altered by a change in renal function.

Starting doses for strong opioids

- *Previously on nonopioid:* 10-30mg daily.
- *Previously on weak opioid:* 30-60mg daily.

- Poor renal function (creatinine >200 mmol/l): halve the above doses or use equivalent of hydromorphone PO or fentanyl SC.
- Previously on strong opioids: see below for equivalent dose of oral morphine. Increase this by 50% if the patient was not pain-controlled.
- For poor hepatic function: no need to adjust doses.

Breakthrough doses

These are usually the equivalent of a 4-hourly dose.

How often?

- **Regular administration is fundamental to good pain relief.**

Strong opioids should be administered regularly since continuous pain requires continuous analgesia. Instant release solutions or tablets of morphine are effective 4-hourly or diamorphine as a continuous subcutaneous infusion. The controlled release preparations of morphine are effective over their dosing times (eg. MST Continus 12-hourly, MXL once daily). Hydromorphone is effective 4-hourly (Palladone) or 12-hourly (Palladone SR). Once methadone has been titrated (see **Drug formulary**), it can also be given 12-hourly. Fentanyl patches are changed every third day.

Dose increases

- **The aim of dose titration is to prevent the pain returning before the next dose.**

Effective doses of oral morphine range from 5mg daily to more than 1000mg daily. Most patients are comfortable on between 60 and 180mg daily. Doses are increased by 50% every third day. In severe pain two or more steps each day may be necessary- only instant-release preparations can be used in this way (Sevredol, Oramorph, diamorphine). Elderly patients, and those with poor renal function, will require smaller increases every 5 days because of M6G accumulation. Methadone is titrated differently (see **Drug formulary**).

Approximate oral opioid equivalents

Opioid	Conversion factor to oral morphine	Opioid	Conversion factor to oral morphine
codeine	0.05	morphine (parenteral)	1.5
dihydrocodeine	0.1	dextromoramide	2
dextropropoxyphene	0.1	oxycodone (oral)	2
oral pethidine	0.1	diamorphine (parenteral)	3
tramadol (oral)	0.2	phenazocine	5
dipipanone (in Diconal)	0.5	levorphanol	5
		hydromorphone (oral)	7.5
morphine (oral)	1	hydromorphone (parenteral)	15
morphine (rectal)	1	buprenorphine	60
diamorphine (oral)	1		
(accumulation of active metabolites of morphine and diamorphine occurs in renal failure)		transdermal fentanyl See **Drug formulary**	
		Shortcut conversion: oral morphine (mg/24hrs) ÷ 3 = TD fentanyl (microg/hr) parenteral diamorphine (mg/24hrs) = TD fentanyl (microg/hr)	
methadone (oral) see **Drug formulary**			

Nonoral routes for strong opioids

There are specific indications for nonoral routes:
- the last few hours or days of life.
- vomiting, whilst antiemetic treatment is taking effect.
- severe dysphagia.
- acute pain, for rapid effect.
- when there is a need for spinal administration.

NB: Unrelieved pain is NOT an indication for parenteral administration of strong opioids

Choosing a route of administration for strong opioids

Clinical decision	If YES → Action
IS PAIN CONTROL URGENT?	• See page 12 for severe pain.
ABLE TO TAKE ORAL MEDICATION?	• Start morphine solution or tablets.
ARE THERE SWALLOWING DIFFICULTIES?	• *If severe:* see **Dysphagia**. • Change to morphine solution or MST-Continus granules as suspension. • Consider: rectal route or continuous subcutaneous diamorphine infusion.
IS NAUSEA AND VOMITING PRESENT?	• Assess cause and start treatment. • Start continuous subcutaneous infusion (check with pharmacist before mixing opioid and antiemetic).
ARE UNACCEPTABLE OPIOID ADVERSE EFFECTS PRESENT?	• Treat adverse effects if possible (see p21). • Consider spinal route: there is a very small proportion of patients on systemic opioids who have an opioid sensitive pain, but are troubled with unacceptable adverse effects. Such patients can achieve relief with combinations of intrathecal opioids and bupivacaine.
IS THERE POOR COMPLIANCE?	• Consider: fear of opioid, poor instructions, misunderstanding of dose or purpose of opioid, refusal (may be due to desire to regain control). • Usually no need to change route of administration.
Parenteral / oral ratios	3mg oral morphine or diamorphine = 1mg parenteral diamorphine

NOTES (see drug formulary section for more details)

Methadone[21, 22] and **dextropropoxyphene** will accumulate with repeated doses.

Conversion to controlled release There is **no** need to give the last dose of morphine and the first dose of controlled release morphine together, ie. no loading dose is required when changing to controlled release morphine.[23]

Parenteral route: the kindest method is a small volume injection through a fine needles. In most patients there is no evidence of a significant delay in the onset of action. There is no evidence that in chronic cancer pain the intravenous route provides more effective analgesia than regular subcutaneous, sublingual or rectal administration.

Rectal route: This route is a satisfactory alternative to subcutaneous administration- hydromorphone and morphine can both be given rectally in the same doses as oral administration (this includes controlled release morphine- MST [24]).

Managing the adverse effects of strong opioids

· **Rapid clinical deterioration due to opioids is rare –
if this occurs see Emergencies: unexpected deterioration.**
· **Tolerance to analgesia is not a clinical problem and psychological dependence is rare.**
· **Many adverse effects wear off within days, but changing to a different opioid may help.**

Adverse effects of strong opioids

Adverse effect	How common?	Dose related?	Tolerance?	Management
Constipation	Almost all.	Yes.	No.	Regular laxative (eg. co-danthrusate)
Nausea/vomiting -via area postrema	28%[25]	Yes.	Yes (1wk)	Haloperidol PO 1.5-3mg at night for 2 weeks.
-gastric stasis	?15%	Yes.	No.	Metoclopramide or domperidone
Dry mouth	40%[26]	?	?	Local measures (see **Oral Problems**)
Sedation	?20% during titration.	Yes.	Yes (5-7 days).	Usually mild and self-limiting. If troublesome, exclude other causes (drugs, hypercalcaemia). If due to opioid consider alternative opioid or spinal route.
Fear of opioid	?10%	No.	No.	Information, reassurance.
Confusion / nightmares -due to sedation	?5%	Yes.	Yes.	As for sedation above.
-due to dysphoria	?<1%	Yes.	No.	Reduce dose, change to alternative opioid, or consider spinal route.
Hallucinations	?<1%	Yes.	No.	Reduce dose or change to alternative opioid, or consider spinal route.
Urinary retention	rare [27]	?	?	Distigmine 5mg before breakfast or reduce dose.
Myoclonus	?5%	Yes.	?	Reduce dose, change to alternative opioid, or consider spinal route.

NOTES

Tolerance: Opioids show 'selective tolerance' [28] Rates of tolerance vary from rapid tolerance to euphoria (1-2 days), slower tolerance to drowsiness (5-7 days), and the absence of tolerance to constipation. Tolerance to sedation may explain why deaths at night are not increased in patients on morphine[29] and why patients on stable morphine doses are safe to drive.[30] Tolerance to analgesia is not a clinical problem, and most patients remain on the same dose for long periods.[31] The need to increase an opioid dose is often because of tumour growth, or because of a new pain that is less opioid sensitive. If the initial dose of opioid does not cause side effects, it can be increased knowing that the patient is becoming tolerant to most side effects, but not to the analgesia.

Respiratory depression is rarely a problem in patients on long-term morphine.[32] The only exception is when pain (a stimulus to respiration) is suddenly relieved by a nerve block without prior dose reduction.

Drug dependence is not seen in patients with advanced disease taking opioids for pain. Psychological dependence is not observed in clinical practice.[33] Patients treated with insufficient or infrequent analgesics will ask for more opioid, but this is simply a just demand for analgesia. On stopping an opioid patients show no evidence of a 'craving' to restart their opioid. Physical dependence does occur but withdrawal symptoms (usually colic, diarrhoea) do not occur with gradual reductions over 5 days. A very small number of patients (<1%) require 2-3 weeks to reduce and stop.

Change of opioid is appropriate if in treating an opioid-responsive pain, adverse effects prevent titration up to an analgesic dose. Alternatives are hydromorphone, methadone and transdermal fentanyl. Cross tolerance may not occur and care should be taken on converting to the new opioid.[34, 35] See p19 for dose conversions.

PAIN:
NOTES AND REVISIONS (regular revision updates available on CLIP update service)

Physical Symptoms

"Until we unravel the myriad of possible interconnections between symptoms, our treatment should be directed at relieving each symptom that can increase the burden of suffering in seriously ill patients."
Norman Desbiens et al [1]

Frequency of symptoms in Cancer[2], AIDS[3] and motor neurone disease[4]

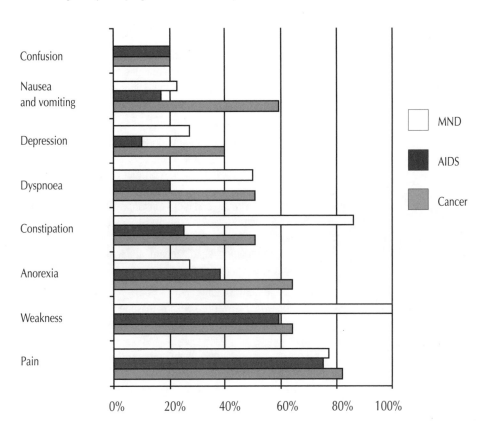

Fatigue and weakness   (64% of cancer patients)[2]

- The commonest symptom in advanced disease.[2, 5]
- Drowsiness, tiredness, lethargy, fatigue and weakness have different meanings for different patients.
- Consider reversible causes (eg. depression).
- Dexamethasone is not first line treatment.

Clinical decision	If YES → Action
IS PATIENT DROWSY?	**Sudden onset** (minutes to hours) **or fast onset** (days)
	• *Respiratory depression or sedation:* see **Emergencies**: unexpected deterioration.
	• *Raised intracranial pressure* (eg. tumours) - high dose dexamethasone + cranial irradiation. If hydrocephalus consider shunt.
	• *Septicaemia-* start antibiotics if appropriate.
	• *Hypoglycaemia* (eg. treated diabetic on little or no diet)- see **Emergencies** (diabetes).
	• *Acute hypercapnia:* if due to inappropriately high inhaled O_2 concentration then reduce O_2 to 24%.
	• *Drugs* (many drugs- check current datasheet) - with opioids wait for tolerance to occur (5-7 days). With other drugs change drug or reduce dose.
	• *Hypercalcaemia* - see **Emergencies**: hypercalcaemia.
	• *Bleeding:* see **Bleeding**.
	• *Hypoadrenalism* (adrenal insufficiency, steroid withdrawal) - hydrocortisone 100mg IV, then maintenance treatment with hydrocortisone (20mg on waking, 10mg at 4pm) and fludrocortisone (100-200 microg. on waking).
	Slow onset? (days to weeks):
	• *Tumour load:* (see notes) - low dose dexamethasone (2-4mg once daily).
	• *Poor quality sleep:* treat cause, consider temazepam 10-40mg at night.
	• *Organ failure* (renal, hepatic) - treat if possible and appropriate.
	• *Hyperglycaemia* (eg. corticosteroids) - see **Diabetes in advanced disease**.
	• *Drug accumulation* (eg. diazepam, antidepressants) - reduce daily dose or change drug.
	Indolent? (months or longer)
	• *Tumour load:* - low dose dexamethasone (2-4 mg once daily).
	• *Hypothyroidism / hypoadrenalism-* evaluate and treat as appropriate.
	• *Loss of sleep:* exclude anxiety or depression (see **The Anxious Person** and **The Withdrawn Patient**.)
	• *Chronic infection despite antimicrobials* (eg. persistent mycobacteria in AIDS): consider low dose corticosteroids in addition to antimicrobials.

Clinical decision	If YES → Action
IS TIREDNESS, LETHARGY, FATIGUE OR WEAKNESS ALL OVER BODY?	• *Infection* (viral, bacterial) - treat with appropriate antimicrobial. • *Anaemia* - transfuse if haemoglobin <10g/dl (full benefit takes 72hours). • *Severe dyspnoea:* see **Respiratory problems**. • *Nutritional deficiency* (iron, magnesium, vitamin B, D)- replace with dietary supplements. Consult dietician. • *Depression or anxiety* - see **The Anxious Person** and **The Withdrawn Patient**). • *Drugs* (many drugs- check current datasheet) - reduce dose or change drug. • *Cardiac failure:* ACE inhibitor, with first dose given as an inpatient. • *Recent surgery:* ensure adequate nutrition. • *Radiotherapy or chemotherapy:* exclude bone marrow suppression. • *Electrolyte abnormalities:* low Na^+ (IADH syndrome, hypoadrenalism, chest infection, diuretics), or low K^+ (diuretics, corticosteroids, vomiting). Treat as appropriate. • *Tumour load* (see notes) - Dexamethasone 4mg once daily, reducing to 2mg after 1 week or medroxyprogesterone acetate 400mg daily.
LOCALISED TIREDNESS, FATIGUE OR WEAKNESS?	• *With proximal motor weakness* consider: Corticosteroids, polymyositis, hypokalaemia, hypo/hyperthyroidism, motor neurone disease, osteomalacia, Lambert-Eaton myaesthenic syndrome (LEMS) [11, 12] • *With any localised motor weakness* consider: Intracerebral cause (cerebrovascular accident, metastases) - if metastases consider high dose dexamethasone + cranial irradiation. Nerve compression - high dose dexamethasone. Cord compression - see **Emergencies** (cord compression). Neuropathy - assess cause and treat if appropriate.
IS THE FATIGUE PERSISTING?	• *Treat coexisting physical symptoms* (eg. pain, dyspnoea, nausea, vomiting) • *Exclude depression or an anxiety state:* see **The Anxious Person** and **The Withdrawn Patient**) • *Modify activities that cause fatigue:*[13] -use rest periods between activities -re-time activities to a time of day when energy is highest -plan regular, gentle exercise -arrange help for low-priority activities. -review sleep behaviours and sleep environment. • *Ensure food presentation encourages sufficient nutritional intake* (see **Reduced hydration and feeding**).

Adapted from Regnard and Mannix [6]

NOTES

Patient perceptions: fatigue is perceived by patients as more severe and persistent than tiredness.[7] Patients describe a number of accompanying sensations: lack of energy, exhaustion, restlessness, boredom, lack of interest in activities, weakness, dyspnoea, pain, altered taste and itching.[7, 8] The concept of fatigue seems to be a combination of physical sensations (eg. slowing up), affective sensations (eg. irritability, loss of interest) and cognitive sensations (eg. loss of concentration).[9] Activity seems to be induced by a perception of loss of control and this complex symptom has far reaching effects which will themselves affect the fatigue and weakness. It can be difficult,

LIBRARY
EDUCATION CENTRE
PRINCESS ROYAL HOSPITAL

however, for patients and carers to differentiate between those sensations and terms are used interchangeably.[10] We have experienced a patient describing 'tired legs' when the problem was motor weakness due to cord compression.

Chemotherapy and radiotherapy: both cause generalised fatigue with peaks 1-2 weeks after chemotherapy.[14] It peaks at the end of a course of radiotherapy,[14, 15] diminishing after 3 weeks.[16]

Drugs are a common cause and can be missed if they accumulate slowly (eg. diazepam with a half life of 23-48 hours) or their rate of elimination changes (eg. the onset of renal failure in a patient on morphine).

Biochemical disturbances: one of the commonest is hypercalcaemia (see **Emergencies**: hypercalcaemia).

Tumour load: humoral factors produced by tumours (eg. tumour necrosis factor) may partly mediate fatigue. Corticosteroids can suppress their production and produce a temporary but worthwhile increase in wellbeing. Patients with cancer are more cognitively impaired than healthy controls.[18]

Chronic infection: end stage AIDS patients may have several organisms or foci of persistent infection (eg. candida, mycobacteria). Corticosteroids are sometimes used with long-term antimicrobials to suppress the symptoms of infection.

Reduced hydration and feeding (64% of cancer patients have anorexia) [2]

- **Consider reversible causes before starting an appetite stimulant.**
- **Reduced intake is normal at the end of life.**

Clinical decision	If YES → Action
IS THE PROGNOSIS SHORT? ie. day to day deterioration	**If hydration or feeding are appropriate:** (eg. thirst, hunger or confusion due to dehydration) • Hydrate and feed for comfort or pleasure (may include IV or SC hydration). **If hydration or feeding are unnecessary** (eg. comatose and comfortable): • Ensure partner, family and staff understand situation. If family or partner feel a need to continue hydration and/or feeding: support family in understanding the situation, but if they remain firm in their belief, negotiate maintenance hydration IV or SC (see notes).
IS THE PATIENT ANXIOUS OR WITHDRAWN?	• Help patient manage anxiety or low mood: see **The Anxious Person** and **The Withdrawn Patient.**
IS IT THE PATIENT'S WISH TO LEAVE THE INTAKE UNCHANGED?	• Ensure good oral hygiene (see **Oral problems**) • Prevent skin pressure damage (see **Skin pressure damage**) • No other action is required.
ARE SWALLOWING PROBLEMS PRESENT?	**Oral phases** (chewing, mixing, moving contents to pharynx): • See **Oral Problems** and **Dysphagia.** **Pharyngeal and oesophageal phases:** • See **Dysphagia.**
IS THE PATIENT WEAK OR DISABLED?	• Regular help with feeding and drinking (ask occupational therapist for advice) • Exclude reversible causes of weakness (see **Fatigue and weakness**). • Treat dyspnoea (see **Dyspnoea**).
IS THE PATIENT CONSTIPATED?	• See **Constipation.**
NAUSEA OR VOMITING ?	• See **Nausea and Vomiting.**

Clinical decision	If YES → Action
IS INFECTION OR ODOUR PRESENT?	• Treat infection with appropriate antibiotics. • Provide adequate ventilation, avoid perfumes (or at least change perfume every few days). See **Malignant ulcers**.
ARE DRUGS A CAUSE?	Reduce dose, change drug, or stop. Consider: • *Drugs causing nausea* (eg. opioids, metronidazole, trimethoprim) • *Drugs causing mucosal irritation* (eg. NSAIDs, chemotherapy, antibiotics) • *Drugs delaying gastric emptying* (eg. opioids, amitriptyline, cyclizine). • *Drugs with central appetite suppressant effects* (eg. opioids, amphetamines).
IS THE FOOD PRESENTATION INAPPROPRIATE?	**Food:** • Ensure the food is presented attractively on small plates. • Keep portions small (have snacks available, use calorie and protein additives that add little bulk eg. Ensure, Caselan). • Vary food (consistency, temperature, taste). • Ask advice from nutritionist and catering staff. **Environment:** Ensure a pleasant atmosphere (coffee or baking smells, company, attractive table cover, alcohol before meals, avoid frying smells). • *If patient is embarrassed* (eg. unavoidable dribbling): ensure privacy. • *If cultural food is required* (eg. Kosher food): ensure this is available.
IS ANOREXIA STILL PRESENT?	• Consider central depression of appetite due to pain (see **Pain**). • Consider altered taste due to Nutritional deficiency (zinc, vitamin B complex): zinc supplement might help.[23] Drugs (phenytoin, flurazepam) Dry mouth (dyspnoea, drugs, radiotherapy, chemotherapy) see **Oral Problems** Related conditions (diabetes, chronic infection, renal failure). • *If all else is inappropriate or fails to improve appetite:* Consider treating empirically with appetite stimulant -dexamethasone 4mg once daily,[24] or medroxyprogesterone 400mg daily[25]
IS THIRST STILL PRESENT?	• Moisten mouth frequently • Consider non-oral hydration: If needed for 3 weeks or less: use IV route or subcutaneous infusion into thighs (see notes). The nasogastric route is a less well tolerated alternative.If needed for 1 month or more: consider percutaneous gastrostomy.[26]

Adapted from Regnard and Mannix [19]

Notes

Deciding to hydrate or feed at the end of life: the decision lies with the patient, with the advice of carers. Every situation is different and fixed policies are indefensible.[20] The traditional view has been that dehydration causes few symptoms at the end of life.[21] There is now a view that dehydration can cause or contribute to an agitated confusional state in some patients.[22] With a short prognosis (day to day deterioration) hydration and feeding should be for comfort or pleasure. Achieving comfort may include treating thirst or an agitated confusional state if these are felt to be caused by dehydration. In patients who are comatose and comfortable, then hydration and feeding are unnecessary. Family, friends or staff, however, may feel a need to continue hydration or feeding in such patients and they will need explanation and support. Occasionally, the partner or family persist with the request for hydration or feeding even though the patient is comfortable. In such circumstances it is reasonable to hydrate since subcutaneous hydration or feeding through an existing PEG tube is unlikely to cause discomfort whilst refusing their request may complicate their bereavement.

Hydration: this is most conveniently done subcutaneously (hypodermoclysis).[27] The antero-medial thigh is the best site in our experience and up to 100ml/hour can be infused without hyaluronidase.[28, 29] Some thigh swelling occurs with volumes above 2 litres / 24 hours, so each leg is used on alternate days. Unlike the intravenous route, subcutaneous cannulae can be left in place for 7-10 days without problems.

Oral feeding: the key is food presentation,[30] with a pleasant atmosphere. Patients may develop taste abnormalities and may prefer sweeter, colder and spicier foods, while others cannot tolerate the bitterness of urea in red meats.[31] An alcoholic drink before meals is more effective poured from bottle to glass rather than dispensed in calibrated plastic pots. The skills of an enthusiastic chef and the advice of a dietician can be invaluable.

Non-oral feeding: the clinical decisions in choosing non-oral routes are in **Dysphagia**.

Taste: 67% of cancer patients in one study described taste changes.[23] They disliked tea, coffee, meat, cheese and spicy foods, but developed a liking for sweet foods. The same patients also had significantly low zinc levels.

Oral problems   (60% of cancer patients)

- **A healthy mouth has an intact mucosa and is clean, moist and pain-free.**
- **Regular mouth care will prevent many oral problems.**
- **Candidiasis and dry mouth are the two commonest problems.**

Clinical decision	If YES → Action
IS ORAL HEALTH AT RISK?	**At risk** (debility, poor oral intake, drugs, local irradiation, oral tumour, chemotherapy). • Twice daily teeth or denture brushing with fluoride containing toothpaste, overnight soaking of dentures, keep mouth moist.

IS AN ULCER PRESENT?	• *Viral* (zoster or herpes simplex):
	oral acyclovir 200 mg 4-hourly for 1 week (400 mg if immunosuppressed).
	• *Apthous ulcers:*
	-topical corticosteroid (triamcinolone in Orabase[35], or betamethasone tablets[36])
	or - tetracycline suspension mouthwash [37]
	(250 mg for 2 mins. then swallowed, 6-hourly).
	• *Malignant ulcers:*
	Anaerobic infection (foul smell)-
	    systemic metronidazole 12-hourly 500mg PO or 1G PR.
	    or 1% topical gel if not tolerated systemically.
	Surrounding cellulitis - flucloxacillin (500 mg PO 6 hourly).

IS THE MOUTH DIRTY?	**If candidiasis is the cause** (white patches, thick debris) : • Start antifungal: ketoconazole 200mg once daily for 5 days. • For longer course or prophylaxis: fluconazole 50mg daily. • *If compliance is difficult:* fluconazole 150mg as single dose. **If no candidiasis:** • Clean tongue: gentle brushing, chewing pineapple (tinned, unsweetened). • Clean mucosa: helped by using a gentle effervescent solution (e.g. 1:1 cider and soda water). • Clean teeth and dentures: twice daily with fluoride containing toothpaste.

Clinical decision	If YES → Action
IS THERE TOO MUCH SALIVA?	• Try hyoscine hydrobromide 75 - 150 microg sublingually 8-12 hourly **or** transdermal patch (delivers ~150microg/24 hours). • Radiotherapy to salivary glands- 1 Gy followed if needed 4 weeks later by a further 1Gy. • *If there is difficulty clearing saliva*: see **Dysphagia**.
IS THE MOUTH DRY?	• Treat cause if appropriate (e.g. dehydration, infection, anxiety, drugs). • Use local measures: -frequent sprays or sips of cold water and petroleum jelly to lips. -ice-cubes, frozen tonic water ± gin, frozen fruit juice, or pineapple chunks. -gently stimulate saliva eg. mints, pineapple or pilocarpine. • Consider: mucin-based artificial salivas- avoid glycerin.
IS THE MOUTH STILL PAINFUL?	**If pain is extensive:** • Analgesia: benzydamine spray (Difflam) or mouthwash (10 mls mouthwash 2-hourly), or benzocaine lozenges (100 mg sucked as required) or Mucaine as mouthwash. • Protection: sucralfate suspension (10 mls mouthwash 4-hourly). • Consider: starting or increasing systemic oral morphine, or consider ketamine. **If pain is localised:** • Topical analgesia: choline salicylate gel (Bongela) (0.5 ml or less topically), • Protection: carmellose paste (Orabase) or carbenoxolone (gel - Bioral; granules -Bioplex). • Exclude candida: a red, painful mouth may be caused by acute and chronic erythematous candidiasis in the absence of white patches.

Adapted from Regnard and Fitton [32]

NOTES:

Oral hygiene: poor oral hygiene may be due to a reduced fluid intake, mouth breathing when asleep and reduced host immunity. A soft toothbrush or sponge will gently clean coated tongues.[33] Irrigation with a warm water or 0.9% saline will help removal of oral debris, and is soothing and non-traumatic. Sodium bicarbonate has an unpleasant taste and may damage the mucosa if it is too concentrated.[34] Effervescent solutions are useful, but hydrogen peroxide foams too rapidly and can damage granulating tissue- cider and soda water in equal parts is an alternative.

Candidiasis: this may present as white plaques (acute or chronic pseudomembranous candidiasis), a red tongue or stomatitis (acute or chronic atrophic candidiasis), leucoplakia (chronic hyperplastic candidiasis), simple inflammation (Newton's type I and II), papillary hyperplasia (Newton's type III), and angular chelitis.[38] With the exception of white plaques, there is no association between oral symptoms and the presence of candida.[39] Cross infection does not easily occur by way of cups and cutlery but may occur by way of carers' hands.[40] Prophylactic nystatin does not reduce the incidence of positive mouth swabs,[39] but in AIDS patients long-term therapy with systemic antifungals may be necessary.

Antifungals: 1-2mls of nystatin must be given at least 6-hourly over more than 5 days to be effective.[41] Ketoconazole 200mg once daily clears 90% of pseudomembranous candida,[42] and is also much more convenient to the patient and cheaper than one week with nystatin. Serious adverse effects with ketoconazole are rare,[43] but there are reports of gynaecomastia[44] and hepatotoxicity.[45] The incidence of potentially serious hepatic injury is very low (1 in 15,000 exposed individuals [46]) and have not been reported for 5 day courses. Fluconazole is effective in a single dose[42] making it useful in patients with a short prognosis, but it is more expensive than other antifungals. Fluconazole is used for longer prophylaxis in AIDS patients with itraconazole as second line.

Pineapple chunks: contain a proteolytic enzyme, ananase, that also cleans the mouth. Unsweetened tinned pineapple is preferable and ananase is still active despite the canning process.

Dry mouth: Glycerin dehydrates the mucosa [47] and should be avoided. Methylcellulose solutions taste 'oily', although this is less with a spray (eg. Glandosane) and a well tolerated alternative is porcine mucin spray (Saliva Orthana). It seems, however, that such sprays are no better than placebo,[48] and frequent sprays with water may be just as effective. The addition of saliva stimulants such as lemon spirit to artificial salivas can cause stinging in patients with ulceration and can exhaust salivary glands. A mixture of glycerin and lemon juice does not improve stomatitis.[49] Stimulants which encourage salivation may help such as pilocarpine[17] (available as Salagen 5mg 8-hourly). Adverse effects of pilocarpine include intestinal colic and bronchospasm.

Oral pain relief: mucosal protection can be offered by topical agents. Sucralfate suspension benefits mucositis due to chemotherapy,[50] and can be of benefit in any painful ulceration. Carmellose (Orabase) paste is an effective protective for local lesions. Local analgesia can be provided by several agents. Benzydamine hydrochloride (Difflam) mouthwash provides local anti-inflammatory action and analgesia for 1-2 hours with minimal numbness.[51] Choline salicylate gel (Bonjela, Teejel) is also effective but can cause pain on application. Mucaine contains a local anaesthetic, while benzocaine lozenges can help acutely painful lesions at the expense of numbness. In very severe pain, systemic analgesia is required. Opioids may provide some relief, but ketamine may have a useful role in this situation.

Constipation   (51% of cancer patients)[2]

- Constipation can mimic some features of advanced disease.
- The need to treat is usually due to a failure in prevention.
- Give appropriate laxatives regularly and titrate to maintain a comfortable stool.
- Diarrhoea can be a symptom of constipation.

Constipation can cause abdominal masses, anorexia, obstructive symptoms, pain, confusion and diarrhoea. Colic with fixed abdominal masses can be mistaken for tumour. Constipation is likely in all patients on constipating drugs and in patients who are immobile, have a reduced fluid intake or are on low roughage diets.

Clinical decision	If YES → Action
OBSTRUCTION ?	See **Bowel obstruction**
HAVE FAECES BEEN EASY AND COMFORTABLE TO PASS?	**If constipation is a risk** (drugs, dehydration, immobility) • Reduce risk: eg. rehydrate, use prophylactic laxatives. • *If stool is infrequent:* this is common in advanced disease, but exclude constipation by rectal, abdominal and, if necessary, X-ray examination.
IS THE RECTUM FULL?	**If faeces are hard:** • Encourage fluids and start co-danthramer or equivalent. • Glycerin suppositories may lubricate to allow easy passage, otherwise use docusate enema to soften stool. **If faeces are soft:** • Stimulate colon with senna or bisacodyl PO (10 hour delay) **If no success:** • Manual evacuation under sedative cover (eg. IV midazolam).
IS THE COLON FULL?	**If colic absent:** • Start regular co-danthramer or equivalent. **If colic present:** • Divide laxative into smaller, more frequent doses or change to lactulose 10-20mls 8-hourly.

CONTACT LAXATIVES: approximate equivalents (based on contact stimulant content only)

  30mls co-danthramer (Codalax) syrup or 10mls co-danthramer strong (Codalax Forte) syrup

= 6 co-danthramer capsules or 4 co-danthramer strong capsules (Codalax)

= 3 co-danthrusate (Normax) capsules

= 10mls senna syrup or 2 senna tablets[52] plus 200mg docusate.

= approx. 10mls senna syrup plus 10mls lactulose syrup.[53]

Typical requirements on 60mg oral morphine daily = 2 co-danthramer strong capsules or equivalent.
Typical requirements on 180mg oral morphine daily = 4 co-danthramer strong capsules or equivalent.

Adapted from Regnard [54]

NOTES:

Constipating drugs include those that reduce forward peristalsis but can increase mixing movements (opioids eg. morphine, diamorphine and loperamide); and drugs that reduce all bowel contractions (drugs with antimuscarinic action, including tricyclic antidepressants, hyoscine hydrobromide or butylbromide, cyclizine, chlorpromazine, methotrimeprazine).

Lactulose can cause bowel distension in higher doses,[55] and in our experience can cause postural hypotension due to fluid shift into the bowel. It has a limited place as an alternative to docusate when danthron (in co-danthrusate and co-danthramer) or senna is causing colic.

Laxative dose titration: proportionately less laxative is required at higher opioid doses. Each patient requires individual titration since the dose range is wide (eg. 1-20 co-danthramer capsules daily).

Patients with **colostomies**: Gently inserting a finger will show if faeces are present. If faeces are present, treat as for faeces in rectum (above). If faeces are absent, exclude obstruction and follow the clinical decisions above.

Paraplegic patients may need regular manual evacuations, but without sedative cover. In these patients evacuation is easier if the faeces are made firmer by using a contact laxative alone (eg. senna).

Respiratory problems   (51% of cancer patients have dyspnoea) [2]

- Dyspnoea can be frightening, and managing the fear is essential.
- Simple measures are often helpful.
- Much treatment is conventional and logical.
- More unusual treatment is available and can be successful.

Clinical decision	If YES → Action
IS PATIENT HYPOXIC?	• Confirm hypoxia with pulse oximeter if available. • Start oxygen (100% via face mask, 24% if previous pulmonary disease with CO_2 retention). • *If gas exchange is poor* (ie. hypoxia persists on O_2): see 'persistent dyspnoea' on p34.
SIMPLE MEASURES?	• Increase air movement over patient's face (fan, open window). • Explain what is happening. • Try sitting patient upright, massage, and distraction.
HAS PROBLEM DEVELOPED RAPIDLY? (minutes to hours)	**Airway obstruction** • Rasping or wheeze from upper airway: see **Emergencies**: stridor. • Oedema of face with distended neck and arm veins: see **Emergencies**: SVCO. • Generalised wheeze on auscultation: start bronchodilator, monitor peak flow. **Dyspnoea due to ventricular failure** • Loop diuretic IV then consider ACE inhibitor for long-term control. • Nurse the patient in a sitting or semi-prone position. **Poor ventilation due to pain** (eg. rib fracture of spinal metastases) • See **Emergencies**: severe pain. **Hyperventilation due to diabetic ketoacidosis** • See **Emergencies**: diabetic emergencies. **Retained secretions at the end of life:** • Hyoscine butylbromide 20mg SC (or hyoscine hydrobromide 400microg. SC if sedation needed) and reposition patient. **Dyspnoea due to intracavity air or fluid:** • *If pneumothorax:* >30%, consider intercostal drainage. • *If pleural effusion:* consider aspiration ± pleurodesis. Consider diuretics (see notes). • *If pericardial effusion:* refer to a cardiologist to consider drainage. **Dyspnoea due to pulmonary embolism:** • Treat symptomatically with oxygen and analgesia (opioids, intercostal block). • Start low molecular weight heparin 2000 - 3000 units SC once daily.[56, 211] Consider referral for a venal caval filter.[57] **If anxiety is present:** • If panic: see **Emergencies**: agitation. • See also **The anxious person**.

Clinical decision	If YES → Action
ARE HICCUPS PRESENT?	• Try simple measures eg. rebreathing from paper bag. • *If gastric stasis or a 'squashed stomach syndrome' present:* start an upper GI prokinetic agent (see **Nausea and Vomiting**). • *If hiccups persisting:* start baclofen 5mg 8-hourly. Increase dose if necessary. [58, 59] • *If hiccups are severe:* try midazolam 2-10mg titrated IV.[60]
ARE AIRWAY SECRETIONS CAUSING DISTRESS?	• Exclude aspiration: see **Dysphagia**. • Start respiratory exercises with physiotherapist if patient is well enough. • *If there are retained secretions at the end of life:* hyoscine butylbromide 20mg SC (or hyoscine hydrobromide 400microg. SC if sedation needed) and reposition patient. • *If sputum is tenacious:* Start regular nebulised saline. Consider a mucolytic agent. (eg. carbocisteine 750mg PO 8-hourly). • *If sputum is thin and loose:* nebulised terbutaline.[62]
IS PULMONARY INFECTION PRESENT?	**If patient is very ill due to advanced disease:** if no symptoms, then no action is required. **For all other patients:** • Start antibiotic: amoxycillin or erythromycin PO (if immunocompromised or this is a persistent infection, send sputum for microbiology). • *For pneumocystis carinii* (PCP) in AIDS start high dose co-trimoxazole (60mg/kg 12-hourly) for 2 weeks, or nebulised pentamidine (600mg daily) for 3 weeks. **For pain due to infection**: see **Pain** p14.
HAS DYSPNOEA DEVELOPED SLOWLY? (days to weeks)	• Exclude ventricular failure, pleural effusion or diaphragmatic splinting (tumour, ascites). • *If anaemic:* blood transfusion if Hb < 10g/dl.[63, 64, 127] Full benefit takes 72 hours. • *If pulmonary tumour present:* start high dose dexamethasone (16mg daily, reducing to lowest dose that will control symptoms). Consider: chemotherapy or hormone therapy if tumour likely to respond. • *If respiratory muscle weakness* (eg. motor neurone disease, muscular dystrophy): refer to respiratory physician for consideration of positive pressure ventilation using nasal or face masks.[65, 66]
IS DISTRESSING DRY COUGH PRESENT?	• Exclude: heart failure, drugs (eg. ACE inhibitors), aspiration. • Humidify room air. Start simple linctus as required. • Lignocaine: 10% spray in single spray to back of throat. Consider nebulised lignocaine (5mls 2% solution over 20mins): patients need to fast for one hour after use. • *If bronchial tumour present:* try beclomethasone 500microg inhaled 6-hourly.

Clinical decision	If YES → Action

IS DYSPNOEA PERSISTING?

Further approaches:
- *If patient is agitated or distressed:* see **Emergencies**: agitation.
- Start opioid: low dose oral morphine.
  Consider diamorphine or morphine nebulised in 0.9% saline.
- Consider nabilone if no cardiac impairment: 100-500 microg PO 8-hourly.[67]
- Consider acupuncture (upper sternum and L14 points in hands) [68]

Plan future support
- Refer to dyspnoea clinic if this is available, [69] and promote 'breathing re-training'.[70]
- Help patient to re-adapt to new respiratory capacity eg. review demands on mobility.

Manage the consequences of dyspnoea
- See **Oral problems**, **Skin pressure damage**, **The Anxious person**

Adapted from Ahmedzai and Regnard [61]

NOTES

Nebulized drugs: the use of mouthpieces is better tolerated and more effective than face masks.[71] Moderate size particles are produced by jet nebulizers and will deposit in the airways. Smaller particles (3-4 μm) will reach the alveoli, but need ultrasonic nebulizers.[71]

Acute hypoxia often results in a marked agitated confusional state and is not always accompanied by cyanosis. A pulse oximeter is invaluable in this situation if available.[72]

Ventricular failure needs urgent treatment even when the prognosis is very limited (hours or days), since the consequent agitation and bronchial secretions will be distressing to patient, family and staff. A common cause is a terminally ill patient being nursed flat when they were previously unable to do so because of breathlessness caused by the failure.

Pleural effusions: if symptomatic these are worth draining, not taking more than 1-1.5 litres at a time. Fluid does not always reaccumulate rapidly- a delay of several weeks is more usual and this may be sufficient time in an ill patient. Occasionally more rapid accumulation occurs, or the patient's prognosis is such that a regular drainage is impractical. Fibrotic agents (of which tetracycline 1G is the least distressing, [73]) are of doubtful value unless a chest drain is used to drain the effusion to dryness. A pleuroperitoneal shunt is an alternative in a patient who is deteriorating slowly (month by month).[74] A loop diuretic / spironolactone combination (as for **Ascites**), is a simple alternative which in our experience helps some patients.

Pulmonary embolus can cause distressing pain and dyspnoea. Standard practice is to anticoagulate, but in patients with advanced malignancy full anticoagulation causes new problems with bleeding or unstable anticoagulation control.[75] In addition, repeated episodes are unusual, but if they occur a compromise is to use low molecular weight heparin which, in low doses, needs no monitoring and can be given once daily.[56, 211]

Respiratory infections: Whether to treat a chest infection in very advanced disease often causes concern. In reality the disease will progress regardless of antibiotics. If the infection distresses the patient (eg. fever, purulent sputum, pleuritic chest pain), and the patient is willing and able to take oral medication, antibiotics are appropriate. In immunocompromised patients reaching the last stages it is necessary to accept that antimicrobials will only suppress an infection. In very ill patients, symptoms can be palliated in other ways: cooling for fever, hyoscine hydrobromide for secretions, analgesics for pain, and corticosteroids to suppress the response to infection.

Opioids can reduce the demand for ventilation without significant respiratory depression. Even with significant pulmonary disease, carbon dioxide retention is unusual.[76] Opioids can be prescribed in the same way as for pain control (see **Using opioids**). If this fails, nebulised opioids have been commonly used, whether or not patient was already on systemic opioids.[77, 78] The basis was the discovery of opioid receptors in the bronchial tree,[79] but there have been conflicting reports as to their efficacy,[80 - 82] Opinion varies from the view that there is a lack of evidence to support their use, [83, 84] to continuing interest in this route of delivery.[71] Morphine is the opioid of choice, but nebulised fentanyl has also been suggested.[71] We have used diamorphine because of its wide availability in a pure, freeze-dried form. Although it does not stimulate opioid receptors, it is easily hydrolysed to morphine. Bronchospasm is a risk with morphine, especially at higher doses of morphine, and one recommendation of good practice is that the first test dose is given where bronchodilator treatment is immediately available.[71] Bronchospasm has also been reported with diamorphine, but in 11 years of use we have never experienced a case of bronchospasm when nebulising diamorphine mixed with 0.9% saline.

Cough: simple linctus or humidified air are soothing preparations that can be repeated as often as required. Bupivacaine given by way of a jet nebuliser through a mouthpiece is helpful to suppress cough arising anywhere down to the larger bronchi.[71, 209] It is not always tolerated and the larger particles may cause numbness of the mouth and throat, preventing safe eating or drinking for several hours. High dose dexamethasone may reduce pleural, pericardial or diaphragmatic irritation by tumour.

Breathing retraining involves helping the patient to readapt to their new respiratory capacity through relaxation, establishing a sense of control, and improving respiratory muscle strength.[70] It has an important role in dyspnoea that persists for several months or more.

Mechanical ventilation at first seems inappropriate in the context of very advanced disease. But for patients with progressive neuromuscular disease, it can significantly improve their quality of life. The techniques are now well established and can improve sleep and daytime symptoms. [65, 66]

Nausea and vomiting   (40% of cancer patients)

- Antiemetic choice depends on the cause.
- A single antiemetic is sufficient in two thirds of patients.[85]
- Any added antiemetics should have a different action.[86]
- Gastric motility disorders have specific signs and symptoms.

Clinical decision	If YES→Action
IS PATIENT MAINLY VOMITING? (ie. little or no nausea)	**Large volume vomiting** (with heartburn, hiccups, fullness or early satiation): • *If dehydrating rapidly* consider total gastric outflow obstruction - will need NG tube and IV hydration for comfort. If tumour is the cause, high dose dexamethasone may help clear the obstruction. • *If not dehydrating rapidly:* this is probably gastric stasis due to drugs (see notes); partial outflow obstruction which may be physical (tumour, hepatomegaly, ascites) or due to disordered motility of duodenum (pancreatic carcinoma); or autonomic failure. Start domperidone (30-60mg PR 8-hourly) **or** metoclopramide (30-90mg SC infusion per 24 hours). Maintain on oral or rectal route. • *If gastric stasis is still a problem*, start cisapride 10mg 8-hourly or 20mg 12-hourly. Consider stopping cisapride and start erythromycin 250-500mg 8-hourly. • *If there is still no improvement:* consider a percutaneous gastrostomy. **Regurgitation** (unaltered food or drink vomited within minutes of ingestion): • See **Dysphagia** . **Distended stomach** ("floppy stomach syndrome"). May contain fluid, air or both. • Nasogastric suction will bring rapid relief, even in unconscious patients. **Compressed stomach** ("Squashed stomach syndrome"). Due to ascites, liver, tumour. Features are the same as gastric stasis but vomits are small. • Treat as for gastric stasis. **Raised intracranial pressure** (may cause vomiting without nausea)**:** see next page.
CHEMICAL CAUSE?	Due to drugs (see notes), uraemia, hypercalcaemia, bacterial toxins. • Low dose haloperidol (1.5-3mg PO or SC once at night).
COULD THERE BE VAGAL STIMULATION?	Due to pharyngeal irritation (candida, sputum), stretched liver capsule by metastases, ureteric distension, bowel obstruction. • Cyclizine (25-50mg PO or PR 8-hourly / 75-150mg SC infusion per 24 hrs). • *If no improvement:* consider second cause eg. chemical cause, gastric stasis.
IS THE BOWEL OBSTRUCTED ?	• See **Bowel obstruction in advanced cancer**.

Clinical decision	If YES → Action
RAISED INTRACRANIAL PRESSURE?	• Cyclizine 25-50mg PO or PR 8-hourly / 75-150mg SC infusion per 24 hours • *If due to cerebral tumour:* start high dose dexamethasone and refer to clinical oncologist for cranial irradiation
IS NAUSEA AND VOMITING WORSE ON MOVEMENT?	**Mechanical distortion of a distended stomach or bowel** • Treat as gastric stasis for stomach or use cyclizine for bowel. **Motion sickness** • Hyoscine hydrobromide 150-300 microg. sublingually 6-hourly. **Other causes** include middle ear infection, vestibular viral neuronitis (eg. zoster), ototoxic drugs, tumour at cerebello-pontine angle, Meniere's disease. • Cyclizine 25-50mg 8-hourly or 75-150mg SC infusion per 24 hours.
FEAR OR ANXIETY ?	• See **The Anxious Person**. • If abnormal behaviour or experience: see **Confusional states**.
IS GASTRITIS PRESENT? (epigastric pain usually a feature)	• Stop NSAIDs. If necessary, restart with omeprazole cover. • Ranitidine 300mg 12 hourly. • Start domperidone (30-60mg PR 8-hourly) **or** metoclopramide (30-60mg SC infusion per 24 hrs). • *If anxiety is contributing:* see **The Anxious Person**.
ARE NAUSEA OR VOMITING PERSISTING?	• Levomepromazine (methotrimeprazine) 5mg once at night PO or SC. May also be given as a continuous subcutaneous infusion. Can be useful if the cause of nausea or vomiting is unclear. • Ondansetron is helpful in a few patients.[95]

Adapted from Regnard and Comiskey [87]

NOTES

Assessment of the cause will depend on knowledge of local spread and metastases, history and examination.[86] Further investigations may be necessary. Commonly overlooked causes are hypercalcaemia, pharyngeal stimulation by copious sputum, gastric stasis and drugs other than opioids. In one third of patients there is more than one cause of emesis.

Clinical features are helpful in some gastric related causes. Large volume vomiting with little or no nausea suggests *gastric stasis*, with accompanying oesophageal reflux, epigastric fullness, early satiation or hiccups. *Total outflow obstruction* produces a similar picture but with rapid dehydration. Symptoms of gastric stasis, but with low volume vomiting, suggest a *'squashed stomach syndrome'* where the gastric cavity is reduced by gastric tumour or by external compression (eg. hepatomegaly). Occasionally gastric tone is absent, resulting in a stomach very distended by fluid, air or both. In this *'floppy stomach syndrome'* only small volume vomiting occurs, with variable amounts of nausea.

Drugs causing nausea and vomiting are numerous. Drugs used in palliative care may cause nausea and vomiting, probably by way of the *area postrema* (digoxin, opioids, phenytoin, carbamazepine, sodium valproate, erythromycin, trimethoprim, metronidazole, baclofen), by causing *gastrointestinal irritation* (nonsteroidal anti-inflammatory drugs, propranolol, ampicillin, long-term antibiotics, cytotoxic drugs, iron supplements) or by causing *gastric stasis* (chlorpromazine, methotrimeprazine, tricyclic antidepressants, hyoscine hydrobromide, opioids, propantheline).

Choosing an antiemetic: The *vomiting centres* can be stimulated directly (eg. radiotherapy), indirectly from higher centres (eg. anxiety) or indirectly through the vagus due to stimulation of the gastrointestinal and genitourinary tracts. A concentration of histamine H_1 antimuscarinic receptors in the vomiting centres[88] is the logic for choosing an antihistamine with antimuscarinic receptors such as cyclizine. The *area postrema* contains the chemoreceptor trigger zone and is stimulated by chemicals such as drugs, biochemical abnormalities (eg. hypercalcaemia), or toxins. A concentration of dopamine D_2 receptors in this area [89] is the logic for choosing a potent dopamine antagonist such as haloperidol. Gastric stasis usually results from delayed emptying due to reduced motility. Metoclopramide and domperidone antagonise peripheral dopamine D_2 receptors, while metoclopramide and cisapride stimulate 5-HT_4 receptors in the stomach and bowel, resulting in more normal gastric and upper small bowel motility. This action also has a role in bowel obstruction.[90, 91] Erythromycin is an antibiotic that also encourages upper bowel motility.[92, 93] Levomepromazine (methotrimeprazine) blocks several receptors including -adrenoreceptors and 5-HT_2 receptors.[94] and has a role in persistent nausea and vomiting of uncertain whose mechanism is uncertain.

Associated management: *Nasogastric suction* is often necessary in total outflow obstruction. In the 'floppy stomach a nasogastric tube can be passed easily (even in semiconscious or unconscious patients) and removed once all the fluid and air have been aspirated. *Parenteral hydration* is needed in some patients (see **Reduced hydration and feeding**). *Percutaneous gastrostomy* is a well tolerated means of giving enteral nutrition when oral feeding is not possible. It may also have a role to play in persistent vomiting due to gastric outlet obstruction, even if this is due to poor motility.[96, 97] *Acupressure* at the P6 acupuncture point on the wrist may have a role in some patients.[98]

Dysphagia
(23% of cancer patients)

= difficulty in transferring food and drink from the mouth to the stomach.
• **Careful assessment may uncover problems with simple solutions.**
• **The advice of a swallowing therapist is invaluable.**

A wide variety of factors can affect the oral preparatory, oral swallowing, pharyngeal and oesophageal phases by altering the anatomy and control of swallowing.[99] Assessment at the bedside will identify problems with the first two phases, but troublesome dysphagia will require specialist assessment.

Clinical decision	If YES → Action
IS THERE DOUBT ABOUT THE NEED FOR HYDRATION AND/OR FEEDING?	See also **Reduced hydration and feeding**. **If prognosis is short** (day to day deterioration) • Hydrate and feed for comfort or pleasure (moistening may be all that is needed). **If dysphagia is due to exhaustion caused by cancer:** • Only consider nonoral hydration or feeding if active cancer treatment is planned.
IS COMPLETE OBSTRUCTION PRESENT?	**If prognosis is short** (day by day deterioration): • Consider high dose dexamethasone if short-term improvement would be helpful. **If prognosis is longer** (week by week deterioration or slower): • Refer for urgent endoscopy. Start hydration and feeding (IV or gastrostomy [26]).
IS ASPIRATION OCCURRING?	In 60% the symptoms are choking, coughing, copious secretions, or frequent chest infections, while 40% can only be diagnosed on videofluoroscopy.[100] • *If tracheo-oesophageal fistula suspected:* refer to surgeons for covered wallstent.[101] • Refer to swallowing therapist for advice.
ORAL PROBLEMS?	• See **Oral problems**
ARE DRUGS THE CAUSE?	• Reduce dose, change or stop drug (see notes for drugs that cause dysphagia).
IS PAIN PRESENT?	• See **Oral problems.**

Adapted from Regnard [102]

NOTES

Swallowing therapist is usually a speech therapist with a special interest. Consider referral if one or more of the following is occurring or suspected: aspiration, prolonged oropharyngeal transit time, and continuing dysphagia despite a normal examination at the bedside. They offer important advice and help in managing dysphagia.

History: localisation by the patient is accurate in most cases.[100] In contrast, difficulties with certain food consistencies cannot be relied upon to indicate the pathology. Symptoms due to aspiration and the site and character of pain are useful.

Drugs causing dysphagia: due to extrapyramidal disorders (antimuscarinic drugs, metoclopramide, haloperidol); increasing lower oesophageal tone (metoclopramide, domperidone), altered upper oesophageal tone (dantrolene), irritating or damaging mucosa (cytotoxics, nonsteroidal anti-inflammatory drugs).

Clinical decision	If YES → Action
IS PHARYNGEAL OR OESOPHAGEAL PATHOLOGY PRESENT?	**Malignancy** (luminal, mural or extrinsic) • Refer to surgical gastroenterology team for assessment (see notes). • *If acid reflux produces tenacious regurgitated material* (due to protein precipitation by gastric acid): start ranitidine. **Infection** • *If candidiasis:* ketoconazole or fluconazole (see **Oral problems**). • *If viral* (eg. zoster, simplex, cytomegalovirus): treat according to local antiviral policy. **Cytotoxics or irradiation** • Mucosal protection: sucralfate suspension 10mls PO, 2-4 hourly [50] • See **Oral problems**. **Neurological** • Consider high dose dexamethasone if nerve compression is suspected. • Consider Eaton-Lambert myaesthenic syndrome (LEMS)- see notes. • *If a pseudobulbar palsy is present* (eg. motor neurone disease): refer to ENT team for consideration of a cricopharyngeal myotomy.[106]
WHAT IS THE ORO-PHARYNGEAL TRANSIT TIME? (normally <1 sec) =time from first movement of tongue to last movement of larynx	**If less than 10 seconds:** • Refer for videofluroscopy: *If less than 10% of swallowed material is aspirated:* refer to swallowing therapist for advice on modifying the swallowing technique. *If more than 10% is aspirated or modification of swallowing is nor possible:* use non-oral feeding as below. **If more than 10 seconds:** Use non-oral feeding: nasogastric tube for 1-3 weeks use, or percutaneous gastrostomy (PEG) for longer use.[26] • Change food consistency to one that patients find they can manage (soft is not always best). • Offer small snacks with nutritional supplements.

Adapted from Regnard [102]

Oesophageal, gastric and intestinal candidiasis:[103] Clinical evidence of oral candidiasis is present in only 50% of patients with oesophageal candidiasis.[104] The radiological appearance on a barium swallow is characteristic.

Dexamethasone is useful in reducing peritumour oedema and may open an obstructed lumen. In head and neck cancer patients they may also improve neurological function when perineural tumour invasion has occurred.

Treatments for dysphagia: *Radiotherapy* can be given as a single intracavity dose -used for oesophageal carcinoma it can relieve dysphagia in up to 54% of patients for a median of 4 months.[107] External beam treatment over several sessions can also relieve dysphagia. *Laser* can be used as first line and has advantages over intubation.[101, 108 - 110] Small, metal stents are increasingly being used as an alternative to intubation.[101]

Test swallow: a crude test swallow can be done at the bedside. A *dry swallow* is done with the examiners' fingers resting lightly on the throat over the thyroid cartilage and behind the chin. The time in seconds is measured from the first movement of the tongue to the last movement of the larynx. This is the oropharyngeal transit time and is usually less than one second. A *wet swallow* is done with 5mls water. Speaking immediately after swallowing will uncover silent aspiration by the 'gargle' quality to the voice, or by coughing.

Nonoral feeding will be necessary in patients for whom other methods are inappropriate, and in those where continued feeding is appropriate. Indications are: long oropharyngeal transit times (diagnosed clinically), in patients who aspirate more than 10% of swallowed material (diagnosed radiologically), and in patients who require more nutrition than they can manage orally. Nasogastric feeding is poorly tolerated by patients even with fine bore tubes.[111] In contrast, percutaneous gastrostomy (PEG) is effective with a low complication rate,[26] and has important advantages over nasogastric feeding.[112, 113]

Eaton-Lambert myaesthenic syndrome (LEMS) is a paraneoplastic syndrome occurring in 3% of lung cancers and occasionally in other cancers.[11] It causes proximal weakness in the legs and occasionally the arms, a waddling gait, together with bulbar symptoms, including dysphagia. Treatment is with prednisolone (60mg or more daily), azothiaprine or IV immunoglobulins and plasma exchange.[12]

Urinary problems   (23% of cancer patients)

Clinical decision	If YES → Action
IS THE URINE NORMAL COLOUR BUT CLOUDY?	• Test for nitrites and leukocyte esterase: a positive result suggests infection. **In the absence of UTI symptoms:** • *If protein present:* exclude protein-losing nephropathy. **In the presence of UTI symptoms:** • *If urine dipstick test is negative:* consider candida.[115] • *If GU tract is normal:* give trimethoprim 200mg 12-hourly for 3 days. Culture is usually unnecessary in females. • *If infection persists or GU tract is abnormal* (tumour, catheter): culture and give 7 day course of a cephalosporin (continue for 4-6 weeks if pyelonephritis is present). • *If an enterovesical fistula is present* (mixed enterococci on culture): treat only if symptoms are troublesome since eradication of infection is impossible.
HAS THE URINE CHANGED COLOUR?	**If positive for blood on testing** • *If bleeding is severe:* insert 24F gauge catheter and irrigate with 0.9% saline to remove clots. Instil with 1% alum solution 50mls for 30 minutes. If this is insufficient, instil 1% alum at a rate of 5ml/hour for 24-72hours. See also **Bleeding**. • Test urine to exclude infection, culture if necessary. • *If the source is unclear:* refer to urologist to consider pyelogram or cystoscopy. • *If tumour is the source:* start ethamsylate 500mg 6-hourly PO (do not use tranexamic acid). Refer to oncologist to consider radiotherapy or embolisation. **If this is not blood** • Reassure patient • Consider other causes of colour change: orange-red (danthron, senna, bile, rifampicin, rhubarb), red-brown (adriamycin, bile, beetroot, food dyes), green-black (mitoxantrone, bile).

Adapted from Regnard and Mannix [114]

NOTES

Urinary tract infections: a crystal clear urine of normal colour that is negative for nitrites and leukocyte esterase is likely to be clear of infection.[116-118] An infection is suggested by cloudiness together with one or more of the following: dysuria, frequency, incontinence, strong smelling urine, pyrexia, loin pain or confusion. When a patient first presents with an infection single dose antibiotics are adequate and culture is unnecessary for most women.[119] 7 day courses are necessary for recurrent infection or if the genitourinary tract is abnormal. Patients with urethral catheters invariably have urine that contains bacteria- treatment is only required in the presence of local or systemic symptoms.

Haematuria: It is unusual for blood loss to be severe, so oral iron supplements may be sufficient to prevent symptomatic anaemia. Often it is the patient's anxiety that is uppermost and reassurance may be the most effective treatment. Infection should always be excluded. Palliative radiotherapy can reduce haematuria arising from a bleeding malignant lesion in the urinary tract. Ethamsylate reduces bleeding by enhancing platelet adhesion and it is useful for sources anywhere along the renal tract since it is excreted unchanged in the urine. Bladder irrigation with a 1% Alum solution can reduce severe bleeding from the bladder.[120] To be avoided are: tranexamic acid (produces very hard clots that can cause obstruction and are difficult to remove), and diathermy (may make bladder bleeding worse[120]).

Clinical decision	If YES → Action
IS PAIN PRESENT?	**Pain in the midline** • *If pain is in the penis or urethra:* test urine to exclude UTI. • *If the trigone (base of bladder) is being irritated* (produces pain felt at the tip of the urethra): -irritation by catheter: reduce volume of balloon or consider intermittent catheterisation. -irritation due to tumour: try bladder instillation of 20mls 0.25% bupivacaine for 15mins. 12-hourly. Consider radiotherapy. • *If pain is felt in the lower abdomen:* this may be bladder irritability or spasm due to- -catheter: reduce balloon volume, consider intermittent catheterisation. -infection: if this is persistent, try instilling bupivacaine as above. -drug-induced cystitis (NSAIDs, some cytotoxics):[121] stop drug. -urinary retention: see decreased urine output (p42). -unstable bladder: see incontinence opposite **Unilateral pain** • *If pain is in the groin:* this may be ureteric colic due to irritation or obstruction. Give hyoscine butylbromide 20mg IV for immediate effect, followed by diclofenac 75mg IM or 100mg PR for control lasting several hours. Exclude stones or blood clots as a cause of obstruction. For obstruction due to tumour, try high dose dexamethasone. • *If pain is felt in the loin:* this may be renal capsule distension or irritation. -infection: exclude TB or pyelonephritis. -haemorrhage: diamorphine 5mg SC if not on opioid, otherwise use equivalent of current analgesia. Consider ketamine (see **Drug formulary**). -tumour: start opioid or increase existing opioid by 50% every 3rd day if needed. If renal function is poor, avoid NSAIDs. See **Pain** -bilateral ureteric obstruction: see p42.

Adapted from Regnard and Mannix [114]

NOTES

Trigone pain: the trigone is at the base of the bladder, surrounding the urethral opening. Irritation of this area can cause pain that radiates to the tip of the distal urethra. Catheter balloons are a common cause and reducing the balloon volume can help.

Bladder pain due to tumour or persistent infection can be eased with local anaesthetic. 20mls of 0.25% bupivacaine are placed in the bladder and left for 15 minutes. This can be repeated using an intermittent catheterisation technique as described in the notes on the next page.

Ureteric pain can be severe (so-called 'renal colic'). Hyoscine butylbromide will provide immediate relief, while diclofenac offers longer term analgesia.

Persistent pain may require ketamine or spinal analgesia.

Desmopressin: a synthetic analogue of vasopressin (antidiuretic hormone). It reduces urinary output overnight and is occasionally helpful in otherwise intractable nocturnal incontinence.[122] A fluid intake/output chart is started, and no fluids given after 6pm. 10 micrograms of desmopressin is given nasally at bedtime. It is important the patient produces a daytime output of at least 500mls, otherwise water intoxication can occur.

Clinical decision	If YES → Action

IS URINARY INCONTINENCE PRESENT?

If a fistula is present (vesicovaginal or vesicorectal)
- Plan regular voiding through urethra and use water absorbent pads.
- Catheterisation may help by keeping bladder empty, but leakage often still occurs.
- *If this is a vesicovaginal fistula:* try vaginal tampons overnight.
- *If nights are disturbed by incontinence:* give desmopressin 10-40 microg. intranasally at night to stop overnight renal production of urine.

In the absence of a fistula
- Exclude overflow due to urethral or catheter obstruction (urge to micturate, full bladder on examination): see decreased urine output on next page.
- *Confusional state causing inappropriate micturition:* see **Confusional states**.
- *Total urinary incontinence* (ie. no control present- usually due to local tumour): catheterisation with long-term indwelling catheter.
- *Stress incontinence* (incontinence on straining): exclude a hypotonic bladder (see below). Otherwise try a ring pessary. Most patients are not well enough to consider pelvic floor exercises or surgery.
- *Neurological* (caused by damage to neurological control of bladder):
  -hypotonic (neuropathic) bladder following damage to sacral plexus or spinal cord compression below T11 (causes difficulty initiating micturition, intermittent stream, incomplete emptying, recurrent infections, stress incontinence): teach intermittent catheterisation.
  -unstable bladder caused by damage to suprasacral pathways (causes frequency, nocturia, and urgency): imipramine 10-20mg at night (may need up to 100mg), **or** propantheline 15-30mg 8-hourly.[123]
  -unsustained bladder due to spinal cord damage or multiple sclerosis (features same as unstable bladder, but symptoms are worsened by imipramine or propantheline); teach intermittent catheterisation.
- *Bypassing catheter:* reduce balloon volume or change to smaller size catheter.
- *Poor mobility:* Supply urinal and refer to physiotherapist. Consider sheath catheter in men, or intermittent catheterisation.
- *If nights are disturbed by incontinence:* give desmopressin 10-40 microg. intranasally at night to stop overnight renal production of urine.

Manage the consequences of incontinence:
- *Skin care:* use dimethicone-based creams to protect skin (see **Skin pressure damage**).
- *Personal hygiene:* provide encouragement and help to wash regularly and change clothes if needed.
- *Poor body image:* see **Anxiety**, **The Angry person**, **The Withdrawn patient**.

Adapted from Regnard and Mannix [114]

Clinical decision	If YES → Action

HAS URINARY OUTPUT CHANGED?	**Increased urine output**
	
	• *Drugs:* usually diuretics- reduce dose or help with regular toiletting.
	• *Endocrine:*
	  Diabetes mellitus: see **Diabetes**.
	  Hypercalcaemia: see **Emergencies:** hypercalcaemia.
	• *Cardiac failure with nocturia:* ACE inhibitor.
	• *Chronic renal failure:* no action is usually appropriate in very advanced disease.
	
	Decreased urine output
	
	• *Dehydration:* may require correction (see **Reduced hydration and feeding**).
	• *Obstruction of both ureters:* Start high dose dexamethasone. If appropriate, refer to the urologists for consideration of insertion of a ureteric stent or percutaneous nephrostomy.[126]
	• *Obstruction of urethra:*
	  -distortion caused by faecal impaction: see **Constipation**.
	  -tumour: catheterisation is usually required.
	  -prostatic hypertrophy: catheter or surgery. Some patients respond to selective selective a-blockers (eg, indoramin), but hypotension on first dose is a risk.
	  -increased sphincter tone caused by antimuscarinic drugs: reduce dose or stop
	• *Obstruction of catheter:* washout or replace.
	• *Endocrine (inappropriate ADH syndrome):* tumours can produce antidiuretic hormone causing fluid overload. Demeclocycline blocks the effect of ADH and is given PO 300-600mg 12-hourly.

HAS URINE FREQUENCY CHANGED?	**Increased frequency**
	
	• *Causes of increased urine output:* see above.
	• *Bladder irritability:*
	  -infection: see p39.
	  -unstable bladder: see previous page.
	  -anxiety: see **The anxious person**
	  -obstruction with overflow: see decreased urine output above.
	• *Small capacity bladder* (due to tumour): regular voiding or intermittent catheterisation.
	
	Decreased frequency
	
	• *Causes of decreased urinary output:* see above.
	• *Antimuscarinic drugs* (eg. hyoscine, tricyclic antidepressants) causing increased sphincter tone: reduce dose or stop drug.
	• *Neurological problems:* see previous page.

Adapted from Regnard and Mannix [114]

Bypassing catheter may be due to a) large balloon causing bladder irritability (reduce balloon volume by half), b) a catheter that is too large stretching and reducing the seal provided by the bladder sphincter (change to a smaller size and always use a 12CH size at first), or c) due to obstruction (washout or change catheter).

Intermittent self-catheterisation is underused and yet is safe, effective and suitable for both men and women. Because the bladder is emptied completely, the risk of infection is reduced in those with residual urine. At least four times a day the following technique should be used during which sterility is **not** necessary:[124, 125] 1) wash hands, 2) wash skin around urethra with warm water, 3) insert 10FG catheter with KY lubricant jelly until urine flows, 4) once urine has stopped flowing gently rotate catheter and when no further urine flows, slowly withdraw the catheter, 5) rinse catheter in tap water and leave immersed in a 0.016% sodium hypochlorite solution (Milton no.1 in 300ml water) for at least 30 minutes.

Urinary retention: Constipation is a common cause of retention in the elderly or debilitated. Morphine is an unusual drug cause of retention and more common causes are tricyclic antidepressants and antimuscarinic drugs.

Sex and the catheter: Some patients and their partners are still able and willing to consider intercourse, but afraid of the catheter. Many women are able to have satisfactory intercourse with an indwelling catheter, although intermittent self catheterisation is a better alternative. Men who are able to achieve an erection can do so with a catheter present. Gentle intercourse is possible with a disconnected catheter (after draining the bladder), and placing a condom over penis and catheter. If the ejaculatory mechanism is undamaged this can still occur with a catheter, but may be painful. Self recatheterisation or a condom catheter are alternatives to indwelling catheters.

Skin pressure damage   (19% of patients)

- Prevention starts with identifying patients at risk.
- Healing is not realistic if the prognosis is short.
- No single agent exists that will clean ulcers.

Clinical decision	If YES → Action
IS THERE A LOW RISK OF PRESSURE DAMAGE?	• Check skin and risk score weekly or more often if the patient's condition deteriorates.
IS THERE A MODERATE TO HIGH RISK OF PRESSURE DAMAGE?	• Distribute pressure: special surfaces or mattresses, regular turning, taking care with positioning. • Prevent trauma to pressure areas: ensure careful handling and lifting by all. • Ensure the skin is kept clean: avoid contact with urine or faeces. • Moisturise pressure areas: daily application of a moisturising cream. • Reassess daily: pressure areas and risk score. Measure or photograph weekly.
IS PAIN PRESENT?	• Topical analgesia: ibuprofen gel or benzydamine cream to ulcer edge. Topical opioid onto ulcer may be an alternative.[128] • Systemic analgesia: oral morphine or consider SC ketamine. • Local analgesia: consider spinal analgesia. • *For pain during dressing changes:* see p15. • *For other pains:* see **Pain**.
IS THE PROGNOSIS TOO SHORT TO ALLOW HEALING?	eg. day to day deterioration. • Treat and mask odour: see **Malignant ulcers**. • Choose dressings for comfort: eg. moisture-retaining dressings, or calcium alginate dressings if exudate is high. • Manage pain: as above.
IS IMPROVING NUTRITION POSSIBLE?	• Maintain hydration and nutrition: especially vitamin C and zinc.[129, 130] Consider advice from a dietician. See also **Reduced hydration and feeding**.

Adapted from Bale and Regnard [131]

NOTES

Assessing risk: a number of pressure sore prediction scores are available such as the Waterlow risk score.[132]

Pressure relief: special mattresses, seat cushions and careful handling will reduce the risk of tissue breakdown. Even using good quality static mattresses can significantly reduce the incidence and severity of pressure sores.[133]

Classifying wounds: colour was thought to indicate the wound condition but this is probably too simplistic.[134] Early damage can be difficult to classify, although one suggestion is that the skin of early damage feels warmer than surrounding skin.[135] Current consensus uses a 0-4 stage classification each with 2-4 sub-categories, and additional categories for the wound bed and infection.[136] Stage 0 = normal skin or damage not associated with pressure damage; 1 = non-blanching discolouration of the skin; 2 = partial skin thickness loss; 3 = full thickness skin loss with some damage to underlying tissues; 4 = as stage 3, but with extensive damage extending to bone, tendon or joint capsule.

The effect of prognosis on management: patients with a short prognosis (day to day deterioration) are unlikely to heal, and even debridement may be incomplete, but odour and pain can be controlled. Slower deterioration (week to week) may allow some healing of shallow ulcers if nutrition is adequate, but only cleansing in deeper ulcers. Cleansing and healing of a deep ulcer will take several months.

Factors affecting healing: adequate nutrition and hydration are two important factors. It is also possible that stress plays a part by delaying healing.[137]

Clinical decision	If YES → Action
IS SKIN SURFACE INTACT, BUT DAMAGED?	• Exclude other causes: infection, malignancy, arterial insufficiency, venous congestion, sensory loss (= grade 0.3) **Superficial damage** (grade 1 or 2) • If pressure care is fully implemented, dressing is not usually required for Grade 1 damage (discolouration of skin). Grade 2 damage with a blister (=grade 2.1) or abrasion (= grade 2.2) may need a light dressing for protection. **Deep damage** • *If hard necrosis* (= grade 3.4.4): hydrocolloid or hydrogel dressing for one week then debride under appropriate analgesia.
IS AN ULCER PRESENT? (Grades 2 - 4)	• Exclude other causes: infection, malignancy, arterial insufficiency, venous congestion, sensory loss. **If ulcer is superficial** (= grade 2.3) • Provide environment for re-epithelialisation: moisture-retaining dressings (eg. Tielle, Allevyn, Lyofoam, hydrocolloid dressings, Op-Site). • Reassess as needed. **If ulcer is deep** (= grades 3 or 4, all categories) • Provide environment for granulation: moist cavity dressing (eg. cavity foam dressing, calcium alginate or hydrogel). For heavy exudate use calcium alginate or cavity wound dressings. • *If bone is exposed:* treat osteomyletis if present and appropriate. • Avoid harmful chemicals: eg. chlorinated solutions (eg. Dakin's). • Reassess daily. **If the ulcer is dirty** (grades 2.3, 3 or 4). • Debride: use hydrogel or hydrocolloid dressings. Use 0.9% saline for irrigation.[139] • Treat and mask odour: see **Malignant ulcers**. • Apply antiseptic: use iodine-based derivatives (eg. cadexomer iodine).[140] • Surgical debridement in theatre may be appropriate in some patients.[138]

Adapted from Bale and Regnard [131]

NOTES

Debridement: necrotic tissue delays healing, produces odour and masks the extent of damage. Dressings that maintain a moist environment remove necrotic tissue without further damage.[141] A hard, dark eschar of dead skin can occasionally prevent access to the ulcer, but the eschar can be softened with moist dressings.

Moist dressings: the ideal dressing maintains high humidity, removes exudate and toxins, provides thermal insulation, is impermeable to bacteria, free from particles and toxins, and capable of removal without further damage or pain.[142] Traditional gauzes, antiseptics and hypochlorites (eg. Milton), do not fulfil these needs.[143] Few trials have shown any one dressing to have an advantage, and choice will depend not only on the type of wound, but also on availability, experience of the carer, the site of the wound, and patient preference or tolerance.[144] Hydrogels (eg. Intrasite gel) are useful where slough and infection are present. Hydrocellular Allevyn or alginate Kaltostat are useful for heavy exudates. Hydrocolloids (eg. Comfeel, Granuflex) maintain a moist environment useful for debridement and healing .

Other dressings: Semipermeable adhesive film dressings (eg. Opsite, Tegaderm) are useful in maintaining humidity in shallow ulcers (<0.5cm) or in protecting very early damage. Silicone foam dressing (Cavi-Care) can be useful in cavities where frequent cleansing is required.

Pain can be eased by applying topical 3% benzydamine (Difflam) cream to the painful areas, covered by a semipermeable film[145] (eg. Tegaderm, cling-film or food wrap).

Malignant Ulcers

- Each malignant ulcer requires individual assessment.
- Healing may be possible, but comfort is the primary aim.
- Malignant ulcers can have a major impact on body image and the ability to cope.

Clinical decision	If YES → Action
IS RADIOTHERAPY POSSIBLE?	• Refer to oncologist. • Do not use metal-containing topical agent (eg. Flamazine) during treatment.
IS ULCER BLEEDING?	• See **Bleeding**.
ALTERED BODY IMAGE?	• Improve cosmetic appearance - camouflage, silastic foam dressing to fill cavities or latex prosthesis. • Enable to cope with altered image - listening and discussion of problems (including sexual). • Refer for counselling or cognitive therapy if necessary. • See also **The Angry person**, **The Anxious person** and **The Withdrawn patient**.
IS IT DIRTY?	See **Skin pressure damage**. See notes below for odour.
IS DISCHARGE EXCESSIVE?	**If sinus or fistula present:** • Reduce volume of discharge: radiotherapy if secretory. Systemic metronidazole if anaerobic infection. Consider octreotide. • Divert discharge: stoma bag if adhesion on flat surface possible. Consider surgical diversion eg. colostomy, urostomy. **If discharge is from ulcer:** • Reduce inflammation: potent topical corticosteroid (eg. Dermovate) once daily for one week. • Absorb discharge: high absorbent dressings eg. hydrocellular Allevyn, alginate Kaltostat. • Protect surrounding skin: barrier ointment eg. dimethicone based cream.
IS PAIN PRESENT?	**Only at dressing changes:** • See **Pain** Clinical decision 4 on p15. **At any time:** • Review systemic analgesia. Consider ketamine (see **Drug Information**) or spinal analgesia.
IS ULCER ITCHY?	• Remove allergen - exclude allergy to dressing or topical agent. • Reduce inflammation - NSAID (eg. ibuprofen or diclofenac) or use topical steroid (eg. Dermovate) daily for 1 week.

Adapted from Saunders and Regnard [146]

NOTES

Odours: attempts to mask a smell with other odours soon fail as the patient associates the new odour with the unpleasant one. Foul odours due to anaerobic infection will often respond to metronidazole 400mg PO 8-hourly or PR 500mg 12-hourly. Topical 0.8% metronidazole gel is also effective,[147] but much more expensive and should be restricted to patients where systemic metronidazole is not tolerated or is ineffective. Other methods include radiotherapy, or cryotherapy with liquid nitrogen since these may reduce tumour bulk and so reduce the amount of dying tumour tissue that predisposes to infection and odour.

Isolating the odour may be possible with charcoal dressings (Actisorb Plus, Lyofoam C) or colostomy bags for fistulae. Oxychlorodene (Ostobon) has no inherent odour and is effective in removing unpleasant odours. It is irritant if directly applied to tissues but can be sprinkled between dressings or into colostomy bags. Hydrocolloid (eg. Comfeel, Granuflex) can slightly reduce odour. Hydrogels (eg. Intrasite gel) help in removing infected slough. Cling film (food wrap) can be placed over dressings to provide an additional barrier to odour.

Fistulae: Try to fit colostomy bags over the fistula -the paediatric types are easier to fit because of a softer flange. Oxychlorodene (Ostobon) will reduce any odour from ostomy bags (see above). If the area around the wound is uneven, the irregularities can be made smooth with fillers such as Orabase paste, allowed to dry and covered with a hydrocolloid dressing (eg. Comfeel, Granuflex).[148] Silastic foam is helpful when it is desirable to reduce the amount of discharge as in external fistulae connecting with the oral cavity. The dressing forms a close fitting, comfortable and washable dressing that reduces fluid loss.[149, 150] Less easily available alternatives are to use a latex mould,[151] or alginate materials normally reserved for dentistry since these are more versatile and longer lasting- any local dental school would advise. A rectovaginal fistula may allow stool to pass vaginally, allowing the stool to become firmer (by reducing the laxative or giving a low dose of loperamide) can reduce the amount passing by way of the vagina.

Skin defects cause problems in fitting dressings or in the cosmetic appearance. Silastic foam or alginate dressings, or a latex mould offer some solutions as described in the note on fistulae.[149 - 151]

Vaginal and rectal discharges due to local carcinomas may become less offensive with antiseptic douches/lavage eg. povidone-iodine (Betadine vaginal gel or douche). Corticosteroids (given rectally or vaginally) will help if local inflammation is present. Regularly changed tampons can reduce vaginal discharges if there is no discomfort on insertion. Perineal and perianal skin often need protection from the continual moisture with barrier creams eg. zinc oxide paste. Referral for radiotherapy, diathermy, cryotherapy is worth considering, **unless** a fistula is present or there is a risk of a fistula developing.

Octreotide is helpful in patients with postoperative small bowel fistulae,[152] and may be useful in other fistulae.

Generalised pruritus (itching)

An attempt to diagnose the cause is an important first step since this may indicate specific treatments, in particular drugs, eczema, infestations, contact dermatitis, iron deficiency and uraemia should be excluded.

Clinical decision	If YES → Action
IS SKIN DRY?	• Avoid: heat, hot baths, rough underclothing, calamine and other drying agents. • Moisturise - aqueous cream to driest areas, bathing oil to bath water.
IS SKIN WET?	• Protect skin folds: barrier cream (silicone based) or ointment (eg. zinc oxide). • Dry skin on exposed areas: use hair drier on the coolest setting or pat gently with towel (do not rub). • *If distant source* (urine, faeces, fistula) - reduce or stop source. • *If excessive sweating:* exclude infection (chest and urine commonest). Consider other causes (anxiety, fear, morphine, malignancy, menopause). - low dose thioridazine may help (10-50mg PO at night).
IS SKIN COLOUR ABNORMAL?	**If paler than usual:** • Consider iron deficiency anaemia (if chronic renal failure consider erythropoietin). **If darker than usual:** • Yellow (jaundice): treat as for dry skin. Exposure to UV light can be soothing. Also consider high dose dexamethasone or biliary shunt. • Red (erythema): consider cellulitis (especially in the presence of lymphoedema), drug reaction, pressure damage, local allergy or atopic dermatitis. • Violaceous, blue or black: consider bruise, skin metastasis, ischaemia.
IS SKIN DAMAGED?	• Exclude infection (candida, scabies, lice), other skin disorders or pressure damage.
IS ITCHING PERSISTING?	• Consider a systemic drug: cimetidine has been used in Hodgkin's[153] and polycythaemia vera,[154] ondansetron in cholestasis,[155] and naltrexone (an opioid antagonist)[156] or erythropoetin[157] in uraemia.

NOTES

Cupitch syndrome[158] (cutaneous pain and itch): is occasionally seen in patients with *en cuirass* breast cancer. The skin surrounding the tumour is often red, painful and itchy and may be due to local prostaglandin production. Both pain and itch may respond to an antiprostaglandin eg. diclofenac or flurbiprofen.

Jaundice: pruritus does not always relate to the severity of the jaundice. Cholestyramine will be ineffective in total biliary obstruction since there are no bile salts in the bowel. In biliary obstruction, high dose dexamethasone (12 - 16mg daily) may relieve the obstruction temporarily.

Topical drugs: corticosteroids can be effective when appropriately applied to inflammatory skin disorders. It is best to avoid topical anaesthetics and antihistamines.

Sweating: Some patients suffer profuse sweating, particularly at night. It may be due to fear or anxiety. Occasionally the malignancy will produce a fever with sweating - measures such as cooling with a fan or sponge are effective. In our experience the antimuscarinic drug thioridazine can reduce sweating.[159] Drowsiness is a common adverse effect, but given once at night for night sweats, this is not a problem.

Bleeding   (14% of patients)

- Catastrophic, external bleeding is uncommon.
- It is often possible to control bleeding.
- Exclude coagulation disorders.

Clinical decision	If YES→Action
IS THERE A RISK OF BLEEDING?	• *If on warfarin:* keep INR to between 1.5 and 3. • *If coagulation disorder* (eg. low platelets): consider treatment • *If rapidly growing and erosive tumour:* keep dark green or blue towel and sedation to hand. Consider referral for radiotherapy or embolisation.

IS PATIENT HYPOTENSIVE?	**If resuscitation is appropriate:**
	• Obtain IV access:
	  -start rapid infusion of 0.9% saline and cross match
	  -start blood transfusion.
	• Find bleeding source: visual, endoscopy or radiology.
	
	If resuscitation is not appropriate:
	• *If patient distressed:* diazepam 5-30mg titrated IV (if IV access not possible give midazolam 5-15mg into deltoid muscle).
	• *If haemorrhage is visible:* (ulcer, haemoptysis, haematemesis) - use dark green or blue towels to make the appearance of blood less frightening to patient, partner or family.
	• Place warm blankets over patient.
	• Do not leave patient unattended.

IS A COAGULATION DISORDER PRESENT?	• Consider: low or abnormal platelets, reduced warfarin metabolism, warfarin displaced by drug, disseminated intravascular coagulation, or severe hepatic impairment. • Treatment can be difficult - the advice of a haematologist is essential.

IS BLEEDING SOURCE EXTERNAL?	• *If vessel can be identified:* apply pressure to stop flow.
	• Promote clotting: apply sucralfate or calcium alginate dressing.
	• Prevent rebleeding:
	  -topical: apply sucralfate under non-adherent dressing (eg. Mepitel). Dressing can be left in place for several days, although re-bleeding may need a daily application of sucralfate.
	  -systemic: ethamsylate PO 500mg 6-hourly or tranexamic acid PO 1G 8-hourly.
	• Consider: radiotherapy, diathermy or embolisation.

HAEMOPTYSIS ONLY?	• *If minor* (streaked sputum): ethamsylate PO 500mg 6-hourly or tranexamic acid PO 1G 8-hourly. • *If troublesome* (clots, anaemia or frequent bleeds): consider radiotherapy, laser, or embolisation.

Clinical decision	If YES → Action
HAEMATEMESIS ONLY?	• Stop gastric irritants eg. nonsteroidal anti-inflammatory drugs. • *If minor* (altered blood or positive faecal occult blood): 2G sucralfate on waking and night. • *If troublesome* (fresh blood, melaena or anaemia)- 2G sucralfate 4-hourly + ranitidine 300mg 12-hourly (or omeprazole 20mg PO daily). NB. if source is non-malignant - refer urgently for endoscopy and surgical opinion.
IS SOURCE THE MOUTH OR NASOPHARYNX?	**If nasal:** • *If anterior:* pack with gauze soaked in 1% alum solution or sucralfate suspension. Refer to Ear, Nose and Throat surgeons if rebleeding occurs. • *If posterior:* refer to Ear, Nose and Throat surgeons for packing under observation + diathermy. **If oral:** • Sucralfate suspension mouthwash.
IS SOURCE THE RECTUM OR VAGINA?	• *If minor* (streaking only): observe and consider pads. • *If troublesome* (clots, frequent bleeds or anaemia) - ethamsylate PO 500mg 6-hourly or tranexamic acid PO 1G 8-hourly. • Consider radiotherapy, topical sucralfate paste or topical tranexamic acid.
IS SOURCE IN A CAVITY?	• *Haematuria:* see **Urinary Problems**. • *Intrapleural or intra-abdominal:* exclude coagulation disorder or trauma. Start ethamsylate PO 500mg 6-hourly.
ARE THERE SEVERAL SITES?	• Exclude - trauma, coagulation disorder, vitamin C deficiency, altered warfarin handling, bone marrow suppression.

Adapted from Regnard and Makin [160]

NOTES

Coping with severe, untreatable haemorrhage: sheets and towels can be placed on the bed to temporarily soak up the blood loss -if available, green or blue towels are less frightening since when soaked with blood they look dark, rather than red. Perineal pads will help with the management of low gastrointestinal bleeding. The patient will feel cold because of the hypotension, and will need warm blankets. Such an event is frightening for the patient who may need rapid sedation intravenously. The touch and closeness of another person is essential. Partner, family and staff will need support after such an experience.

Radiotherapy should always be considered for bleeding due to malignancy, especially if the source is superficial. It is helpful in 75% of patients with haemoptysis and will also palliate haematuria. External beam sources are tolerated less well in some areas such as the perineum where even palliative doses can produce troublesome skin reactions in a debilitated patient. Single treatments are possible in frail patients, but internal sources (brachytherapy) are being used to avoid some of these problems. Oesophageal and bronchial sites can be treated with intraluminal sources in a single session. Intravaginal and intrauterine sources can also be used to control bleeding from advanced gynaecological tumours.

Pharmacological agents: drugs can be used topically or systematically:

Topical drugs: Aluminium astringents (1% alum solution, sucralfate) act by stimulating the extrinsic coagulation pathway, preventing fibrin removal and forming a non-absorbent protective layer.[161, 162] Sucralfate alone is useful in controlling the bleeding from a gastric carcinoma,[163] or it can be applied directly to the bleeding point if this is visible. A 1% alum solution has been used to treat bladder haemorrhage (see **Urinary problems**).[120] Topical tranexamic acid is helpful for bleeding from a rectal carcinoma and other tumour-related bleeding.[164, 165] Vasoconstrictors such as adrenaline, have no advantages over these other drugs since re-bleeding occurs rapidly. Sclerosing agents (phenol, silver nitrate, formalin) should be avoided since they cause tissue damage and may encourage further bleeding.

Systemic drugs: tranexamic acid inhibits the breakdown of fibrin clots and is well absorbed orally, but should be avoided in haematuria since it produces hard clots that are difficult to remove and can cause obstruction. Ethamsylate enhances platelet adhesion, can safely be used in haematuria and has fewer adverse effects than tranexamic acid.

Dressings: some such as calcium alginate are haemostatic, acting as a matrix for coagulation and enhancing the intrinsic and common coagulation pathways. Dressings with very low adherence (eg. Mepitel) are useful as a base for applying sucralfate. These and moist environment dressings (alginate, hydrogels) can be left in place for up to 7 days, avoiding any disturbance to the fragile bleeding surface. Cellulose-based dressings should be avoided since they inhibit healing and can cause local reactions.

Heat and cold: lasers can palliate fungating tumours. They can also be used with bleeding tumours within the bronchial or gastrointestinal tract in areas accessible by an endoscope, but there is a small risk of perforation. Diathermy can be helpful, but can make bladder bleeding worse.[120] Cryotherapy may help in accessible sites but the resultant tissue damage later breaks down to cause further bleeding.

Embolisation: can be useful in controlling bleeding,[166] and it has been used in haemoptyses, and bleeding from the bladder,[167] prostate[168] and malignant ulcers.[169] Pain and pyrexia may occur for a few days after embolisation. There are risks, especially in the presence of abnormal anatomy,[170] and the decision to embolise should only be taken with the advice of a radiologist and clinician experienced in the procedure.

Coagulation disorders can be caused by platelet deficiency or malfunction, by excessive clotting (eg. with pancreatic carcinoma), or due to widespread microvascular clotting which uses up clotting factors, resulting in a coexistent tendency to bleed (disseminated intravascular coagulation- DIC). Platelet transfusions are straightforward, but their effect is usually short-lived. Adequate treatment for DIC requires a delicate balance between anticoagulation and encouraging clotting by replacing clotting factors- if treatment is appropriate this invariably requires admission to hospital under the care of a haematology team. In very advanced disease such treatment is not usually appropriate, but some cases of DIC respond to a simpler regimen of an antifibrinolytic such as tranexamic acid and low dose heparin.[171] The advice of a haematologist remains essential. Fortunately such events are uncommon, and usually occur in the last hours or days of life when distressing bleeding can be managed as described opposite.

Oedema

- Stockings are a simple treatment for simple (low protein) oedema.
- Lymphoedema (high protein oedema) cannot be squeezed out.
- The cornerstones to care are SETS
  (Support and compression, Exercise, Truncal massage and Skin care).

Clinical decision	If YES→Action
IS ARTERIAL INSUFFICIENCY PRESENT?	• Measure posterior tibial and **both** brachial arterial systolic pressures with Doppler. • Calculate ankle / brachial (AB) ratio (use highest of the two brachial pressures).[172] *If ratio >1 without insufficiency signs or symptoms:* treat as normal. *If ratio between 0.8 and 1:* use only low pressure support (<30mmHg). *If ratio <0.8:* avoid all external pressure.
IS INFECTION PRESENT?	**If cellulitis present** (limb temperature normal or raised, occasionally local pain): • Start penicillin V **or** erythromycin 500mg 6-hourly for 2 weeks -treat any focus of infection (eg. antifungal for tinea pedis, potassium permanganate soaks for infected eczematous reactions). -if no improvement after 3 days, add flucloxacillin 500mg 6-hourly. **If this is recurrent cellulitis** • Treat as above then continue maintenance of penicillin V or erythromycin once daily for 3 months. • Prevent infection by avoiding skin trauma and promptly treating broken areas.

Clinical decision	If YES → Action
VENOUS OBSTRUCTION?	• *Peripheral thrombosis:* anticoagulate and wait 8 weeks before applying compression. • *Vena caval obstruction:* support bandaging or hosiery can be used, but avoid compression pumps.
IS THIS A LOW PROTEIN OEDEMA?	eg. dependency, heart failure, low albumin **If the skin is good condition:** • Low pressure support (10-30mmHg) eg. Duomed class I or II. • Treat primary cause.
IS THE PROGNOSIS SHORT?	**If the prognosis is too short to allow reduction in oedema** (week to week or day to day deterioration): • Use massage and support bandaging or hosiery (see opposite). • Active or passive movement for stiff joints. • If tumour is compressing or blocking lymphatics: consider high dose dexamethasone (16mg daily).
IS OEDEMA LIMITED TO THE TRUNK, HEAD OR GENITALIA?	• Massage the trunk at least three times daily, plus: -for head oedema: sleep propped upright with pillows. -for abdominal oedema: use support garment (eg. Tupipad lumbar) if genitals free of oedema. -for oedema of the genitals and perineum: use made to measure compression pants, tights or scrotal support.
CAN HOSIERY BE FITTED?	**If skin is intact and limb is a normal shape:** • Fit compression hosiery: see notes. • Encourage normal limb movements and advise on skin care. • Review regularly (initially monthly, then yearly). *NB. Do not use hosiery if the following are present:* severe ventricular failure, AB ratio less than 0.8, sensation is absent, any microcirculatory problems (vasculitis, diabetes), or within 8 weeks of a venous thrombosis.
IS BANDAGING INDICATED?	**If skin is damaged, hosiery has failed, or hosiery cannot be fitted because the limb is too large, too painful or has an abnormal shape:** • Refer to a lymphoedema clinic who will advise on massage, compression bandaging (single layer if shape is normal, otherwise multilayer), exercise and skin care. *NB. They will also advise on the use of bandages if the following are present:* severe ventricular failure, AB ratio less than 0.8, sensation is absent, or within 8 weeks of a venous thrombosis.

Adapted from Badger and Regnard [173]

NOTES

Oedema:

Low protein oedema is caused by water accumulation (eg. ventricular failure), reduced venous return (venous thrombosis, venous insufficiency, vena caval obstruction) or reduced osmotic pressure due to reduced intravascular protein (eg. protein losing nephropathy, malnutrition). This oedema pits easily and fluctuates with posture. The skin is pale and cold, except in venous obstruction when it is dusky, warm and may ulcerate.

High protein oedema (lymphoedema) lymphatic obstruction pits with difficulty, has deep skin folds and changes very little with posture. The skin is pale and cool except in cellulitis when it may be a normal colour or red. In time the skin will thicken and, in the legs, will prevent the examiner from being able pick up a skin fold over the dorsum of the second toe (Stemmer's sign). Eventually warty tags can develop that can leak and become infected.

Mixed: Limited mobility (eg. dependency, paraplegia) produces a mixed picture due to a combination of reduced lymphatic and venous return. In time however, many lymphatic and venous problems show a mixed picture.

Cellulitis produces subtle signs. The skin may look and feel normal (when it should look pale and feel cold) and, without venous problems, any warm area suggests cellulitis.

Lipodermatosclerosis presents as a brawny, wooden area and is due to lymphatic and venous obstruction. It may be mistaken for cellulitis but the treatment is the same as for lymphoedema and antibiotics are unnecessary.

Principles of care: SETS

Support and compression: *Support bandages* provide an outer layer ojflow pressure, low stretch material against which the tissues can push and is used to prevent recurrence of oedema or when a reduction in the limb size is not expected. *Compression bandaging or hosiery* applies elastic pressure to the limb and is used in the initial stages of reducing the limb size. In reality, compromises between these two methods have to be used because of the limitations of bandaging and hosiery. A wide range of *hosiery* is available with two compression classes for arms and three classes for legs. Class 1-3 stockings for legs are available on prescription (eg. Duomed), but higher compression stockings (eg. Medi Forte) have to obtained through hospitals or lymphoedema clinics. Tubular supports, shaped or not, should not be used since they often roll down at one end to form a tourniquet effect. Made to measure hosiery is not used routinely but has a place in abnormally shaped limbs or trunks. Garments need only be worn during the day and can be taken off at night. *Bandages* should be applied by those experienced or trained in their use, particularly as there has to be an understanding about the compromise between support or compression. Bandages are worn continuously, and reapplied once a day- usually this is only necessary for 2 weeks.

Exercises: normal use should be encouraged, ideally while wearing support or compression. Any exercise should be gentle, and are described in a patient information booklet.[174] Elevation hinders movement and should be avoided unless this is the only way to obtain comfort.

Truncal massage is by hand or using an electrical hand massager.[174] It is based on the principles of manual lymph drainage, but is done by the patient or partner and does not depend on the therapist. The basic principle is to clear the way ahead, so that the massage always begins in a healthy quadrant of the trunk, before moving gradually to the affected side.[175, 176] No talc or oil is necessary and it consists of gentle circular motions. Massage takes 15 mins. twice daily and ends with a breathing exercise.[174]

Skin care is essential to prevent a portal of entry for cellulitis. This includes protection (eg., gloves while gardening), prompt cleansing of wounds and moisturising at night.[173, 174]

Compression pumps have a very limited place in the management of lymphoedema. They are powered from the mains and intermittently pump up an inflatable sleeve that surrounds the limb. Because they squeeze fluid into trunk quadrants that are already overloaded, they are only used during intensive treatment that is accompanied by regular massage, and compression. Pressures should not be above 60mmHg.

Bowel obstruction in advanced cancer

(3% of all cancer patients: 10% of those with Ca colon, 25% of those with Ca ovary)

Clinical decision	If YES → Action
IS THERE DOUBT THIS IS A BOWEL OBSTRUCTION?	• Consider other causes of -nausea and vomiting -abdominal distension (eg. ascites) -colic (eg. contact stimulant laxatives) -altered bowel habit (eg. constipation)
IS CONSTIPATION THE CAUSE?	Bowel history, examination and plain abdominal X-ray will help in deciding. • Clear rectum and start laxative (see **Constipation**).
IS A PHYSICAL BLOCKAGE ABSENT OR UNLIKELY?	**Peristaltic failure** (reduced bowel sounds, distension, passing flatus): Exclude peritonitis, septicaemia or recent cord compression • Stop - antiperistaltic drugs (eg. antimuscarinics) - osmotic laxatives. • Start docusate 100mg 8-hourly. • Start metoclopramide SC infusion 30-90mg per 24 hours **or** cisapride (10mg PO 8-hourly **or** 30mg PR 8-hourly).
IS THIRST PRESENT?	Hydrate IV or SC (see **Reduced hydration and Feeding**)
IS SURGERY POSSIBLE?	Surgery is possible if • Patient agrees. • Patient is in good or reasonable nutritional and medical condition. NB. Prognosis is poor if there are abdominal masses or ascites, previous abdominal radiotherapy, multiple blockages, or a small bowel blockage.

Adapted from Regnard [177]

NOTES

In patients unsuitable or unfit for surgery, the traditional 'drip and suck' (intravenous hydration and nasogastric suction) will fail to control obstructive symptoms in approximately 90% of patients.[178, 179] Medical management will keep the majority of inoperable patients free of nausea and pain. Short episodes of vomiting are tolerable if antiemetics have stopped persistent nausea. In obstructions distal to the upper small bowel, sufficient fluid is absorbed to prevent significant dehydration. It is possible to manage patients with complete small bowel obstruction for several weeks in this way achieving a comfortable phase with the option of doing this at home.

Causes of obstruction: *Recurrent abdominal cancer* can cause multiple malignant blockages,[180] especially in ovarian carcinoma where the small bowel is often involved.[181] *Metastatic obstruction* from outside the abdomen is most commonly from melanoma, breast or lung.[182] *Constipation* can cause distension, obstructive symptoms and persistent abdominal masses. A supine abdominal X-ray will differentiate constipation from other causes of obstruction. *Benign adhesions* may occur in up to 20% of patients with recurrent abdominal cancer.[183] *A new primary tumour* can be the cause of obstruction in nearly 10%.[178] *Motility disorders* can cause the same features as a physical blockage.[180]

Surgery: this should always be considered since it may only entail forming a loop colostomy or dividing adhesions, but surgery can have a significant mortality and morbiity.[180] An understanding surgical opinion can be helpful, although it can be difficult to decide if there is a single level obstruction that is amenable to surgery.

Colic can radiate to a variety of sites in the abdomen and elsewhere, but the pain retains the usual pattern for colic recurring regularly every few minutes. In a few patients the bowel can go into spasm, giving a pain that can last for an hour or more, but like colic, is relieved by hyoscine. Hyoscine butylbromide causes fewer central adverse effects than hyoscine hydrobromide. Controlling colic in complete, inoperable obstruction is straightforward since the risk of producing an ileus with hyoscine is not relevant. In partial obstruction it is necessary to preserve bowel motility and yet prevent colic without allowing constipation to develop, which could create a complete obstruction. The use of a laxative with minimal stimulant activity (docusate) with the careful use of antispasmodics (eg. no more than 900 microg. hyoscine hydrobromide sublingually in 24 hours) will enable adequate control of symptoms.

Clinical decision	If YES → Action
IS NAUSEA AND/OR VOMITING PRESENT?	• Start cyclizine (50mg PO or PR 8-hourly/ SC infusion 150mg per 24 hrs) (start at half these doses for patients >70 years age). **If nausea and/or vomiting persist:** • *If obstruction is complete and continuous:* **add** haloperidol (3mg PO or 2.5mg SC at night). • Consider: replacing cyclizine with levomepromazine (methotrimeprazine) 5-25mg SC once at night. Alternatives are: hyoscine butylbromide SC infusion 60-120mg per 24 hrs), or octreotide SC infusion 100-600 microg. per 24 hrs.[184] • *If vomiting persists* (high obstruction, faecal or faeculant vomiting): consider a nasogastric tube or a venting gastrostomy.
IS OBSTRUCTION COMPLETE AND CONTINUOUS?	• Stop all laxatives. Treat a dry mouth (see **Oral problems**). • *If colic is present:* start hyoscine butylbromide SC infusion 60-120mg per 24hrs. • Hydrate and feed orally, using occasional, small snacks. • Consider high dose dexamethasone (16mg daily) if short term relief of obstruction is appropriate.
IS OBSTRUCTION PARTIAL OR INTERMITTENT?	• Stop osmotic and contact laxatives. • Start docusate 100-300 mg PO 8-hourly and titrate to produce a comfortable stool without colic. • Avoid high roughage foods (eg. peas). Continue oral feeding and hydration in small, frequent snacks. • For intermittent colic use hyoscine hydrobromide 75-300 microg. sublingually (max. 900 micrograms in any 24 hour period).

Adapted from Regnard [177]

Proximal obstructions: these are more likely to cause vomiting, but less likely to cause distension. In pancreatic carcinoma most are due to poor motility rather than a physical obstruction.[185] Consequently they cause gastric stasis and can be treated initially in the same way (see **Nausea and vomiting**). If a physical obstruction is present, patients may need gastric aspiration to reduce vomiting and IV hydration to prevent thirst. Some will respond to high dose dexamethasone, but occasionally nasogastric suction or a gastrostomy is needed.[185]

Nausea will respond to cyclizine in the majority of patients. Vomiting may remain but at a reduced volume or frequency and patients perceive it as much less distressing than constant nausea. Vomiting is less of a problem in more distal obstructions. Nauseated patients with distended colons often require the addition of haloperidol, since bacterial toxins are now adding to the nausea by acting on the area postrema .

Feeding and hydration: Most patients will absorb sufficient fluid from their upper gut to prevent symptomatic dehydration. Parenteral feeding is not necessary, unless it is a preliminary to surgery. Patients with repeated vomiting or high obstructions proximal to the mid-jejunum will need intravenous hydration to offset the thirst resulting from the rapid dehydration. As patients deteriorate their fluid intake reduces, and parenteral hydration is not usually needed (see **Reduced hydration and feeding**).

Nasogastric tubes fail to control the symptoms of obstruction in at least 86% of patients.[179] Nasogastric suction or drainage has a place in faeculant or faecal vomiting. Faeculant vomiting is not the vomiting of faeces, but of small bowel contents colonised by colonic bacteria in obstructions lasting a week or more. True faecal vomiting is much less common and is due to a gastro-colic fistula. These types of vomitus are malodorous and distressing for the patients and warrant nasogastric suction, although a gastrostomy is a better alternative if aspiration is needed for more than 2 weeks.

Ascites
(6% of cancer patients)

- **Paracentesis offers immediate relief but poor long-term control.**
- **Combination diuretics offer useful long-term control in some patients.**

The commonest causes for malignant ascites are primary tumours of breast, ovary, colon, stomach, pancreas and bronchus. Nearly one third of the primary tumours lie outside the abdomen. Symptoms include abdominal distension or pain, a 'squashed stomach syndrome', oedema (legs, perineum or lower trunk), and dyspnoea due to diaphragmatic splinting.

Clinical decision	If YES → Action
IS THERE DOUBT THIS IS ASCITES?	Signs of ascites: flank dullness, shifting dullness, fluid thrill. • Exclude: other causes of abdominal distension such as bowel obstruction, abdominal tumour or hepatomegaly.
IS PROGNOSIS SHORT? (day to day deterioration)	**If free of symptoms:** No further action required. **Treat symptoms if troublesome:** • Nausea and vomiting: see **Nausea and vomiting** • Abdominal stretch pain: paracetamol or diclofenac. Try TENS. Consider morphine • Peripheral oedema: see **Oedema**. • If dehydrated and/or hypotensive: rehydrate with colloid or albumin.
IS DISTENSION CAUSING DISTRESS?	• *If dehydrated, hypotensive or the ascites is due to cirrhosis:* -start IV infusion of Dextran 70. **In the *absence* of gross bowel distension or abdominal tumour:** • Carry out therapeutic paracentesis (see notes for details): -drain 2 litres over 1 hour, then drain up to a further 3 litres over 24 hours. -remove tube and place ostomy bag over puncture site. -if hypotension develops start IV infusion albumin. • *If no fluid is obtained:* the ascites may be loculated. Arrange for drainage under ultrasound control. • *If ascites is too viscous to drain* (eg. ovarian carcinoma): consider paracentesis with suction. Alternatively ask surgeon to form an artificial fistula (see notes).
CAN PATIENT TOLERATE DIURETICS?	**For patients able to take oral medication and with good renal function:** • Measure abdominal girth at a marked site each week. • Start spironolactone 100 mg PO once daily. Increase by 100mg every third day up to 200mg 12-hourly. [185, 186] • *If no reduction in girth (or girth increasing):* add frusemide 40mg daily. Patients with peripheral oedema may tolerate doses up to frusemide 80mg + spironolactone 200 mg 12 -hourly for a limited period.[187] • *If hypotension develops:* start IV infusion albumin and reduce diuretic dose. Check serum electrolytes weekly. Continue diuretics at lowest dose that will control symptoms. **NB.** For patients with poor renal function, avoid diuretics (use paracentesis to drain sufficient for comfort).

Clinical decision	If YES → Action
IS A PERITONEOVENOUS SHUNT APPROPRIATE?	**If recurrent ascites despite diuretics:** • Contact surgeons for assessment of shunt insertion. **If patients too ill for shunt placement:** • Palliate symptoms as shown opposite.

Adapted from Regnard and Mannix [188]

NOTES

Types of ascites: Four types can be identified.[189, 190]

Raised hydrostatic pressure: caused by cirrhosis, congestive heart failure, inferior vena caval obstruction and hepatic vein occlusion.

Decreased osmotic pressure: caused by protein depletion (nephrotic syndrome, protein losing enteropathy), reduced protein intake (malnutrition) or reduced production (cirrhosis).

Fluid production exceeding resorptive capacity: caused by infection or neoplasms.

Chylous: due to obstruction and leakage of retroperitoneal lymphatics draining the gut.

Paracentesis:

Equipment: this is best using a peritoneal dialysis (PD) catheter- designed for use in dry abdomens they are less likely to puncture bowel or enter vascular tumour. The PD catheter connects to a standard PD collection bag or can be connected to a urine collecting bag using the barrel of a 5ml syringe.

Local anaesthesia: The use of 0.5% bupivacaine as local anaesthetic for the puncture site allows pain-free drainage for up to 8 hours if necessary.

Puncture sites should be away from scars, tumour masses, distended bowel, bladder liver or the inferior epigastric arteries that run 5cms either side of the midline in the anterior abdominal wall. The best sites are in the left iliac fossa (at least 10cms from the midline) and in the midline suprapubically (the bladder must be empty). A lateral approach is advisable in patients with distended bowel- marked distension is a contraindication to paracentesis.

Drainage: It is possible to drain 5 litres over 24 hours and for many patients with malignant ascites this gives good relief. Patients with other causes of ascites can have much larger volumes that need to be drained over several days. After removal of the catheter any leakage of ascites from the puncture site is collected with a colostomy bag. Leakage usually stops after 2-3 days and so the patient is spared a suture.

Dehydration and/or hypotension: Any dehydration before the procedure, or hypotension during the paracentesis, requires an IV infusion of colloid to prevent further hypotension- Dextran is much cheaper than albumin and as effective.[191] These problems are less likely in patients with peripheral oedema. Cirrhotic patients undergoing drainage of more than 5 litres will need an infusion of albumen (8g/l of ascites drained) or a synthetic gelatin such as Dextran.[210]

Diuretics: spironolactone ± a loop diuretic is well established in the management of ascites related to hepatic disease,[189, 210] but it had been believed that malignant ascites was unresponsive to diuretics. The finding of increased renin and sodium retention in malignant ascites prompted the successful use of spironolactone.[192] The addition of an oral loop diuretic increases the diuresis,[193] although reduction of the ascites is as much due to redistribution of fluid as by diuresis.[194] Case reports on the use of diuretics in malignant ascites continue to appear.[195] In cirrhosis, diuretics and salt restriction are the mainstay of treatment.[210] Whatever the cause of the ascites, however, diuretics can cause electrolyte disturbances and need to be used with caution in patients with poor renal or hepatic function.

Peritoneovenous shunt: Insertion of a shunt requires only a short general anaesthetic and causes fewer problems in cancer than for ascites due to benign liver disease.[196] In advanced cancer there is no evidence that increased metastatic disease occurs following such a procedure.[197] Insertion is easier with a tense ascites since this encourages drainage. The procedure takes 30-60 minutes and can be done under a local anaesthetic. Thereafter inspiratory exercises are used to further encourage drainage (eg. sucking through the nozzle of a 10ml syringe).

Other treatments: in malignancy, systemic or intraperitoneal chemotherapy have been used, while other treatments include intraperitoneal injection of radiocolloids or special strains of *Streptococcus*.[189] The availability of these treatments is limited and often not suitable for patients with advanced disease.

Diarrhoea

(4% of patients)

Clinical decision	If YES → Action
IS PATIENT DEHYDRATED?	**If hydration is appropriate:** • Oral rehydration formula (eg. WHO formula) (oral/nasogastric) or Ringer lactate solution (intravenous). If dehydration moderate to severe use 2-3 litres in first 6 hours, followed by 6-8 litres per 24 hours as long as loss continues.
IS DIARRHOEA INTERMITTENT?	• Exclude: spurious diarrhoea (due to constipation), partial bowel obstruction, food intolerance (lactose, gluten), irritable colon, anxiety and fear. • Exclude infection: culture stool if diarrhoea persists after 5 days or contacts are also affected by diarrhoea. **If bouts severe:** • Consider carcinoid or infection (see notes on p60). **If high osmotic load:** • *Nasogastric feeding:* dilute feeds or increase length of feeding time. • *Gastric dumping* (post gastrectomy): small, frequent snacks. If severe, consider octreotide (see notes).
ARE STOOLS DARKER THAN USUAL?	**If faecal occult blood test negative:** • Consider: oral dye (beetroot, danthron) or iron supplements-reassure patient. **If faecal occult test positive** • *Upper gastrointestinal blood loss:* H$_2$ blocker or omeprazole if peptic ulceration. Use sucralfate if due to gastric tumour[163] or tranexamic acid if due to small bowel tumour.
ARE STOOLS PALER THAN USUAL?	**If steatorrhoea** (pale, malodorous stools that are difficult to flush away): • Loperamide (2 mg with each loose stool, up to 16mg daily) plus: *Pancreatic insufficiency:* enteric coated pancreatin supplement + ranitidine + dietary supplements. *Obstructive jaundice:* ranitidine + enteric coated pancreatin and consider high dose dexamethasone, bypass surgery or endoscopic stent. *Zollinger Ellison syndrome:* high dose ranitidine or omeprazole. *Post intestinal surgery:* see next clinical decision.
HAS THERE BEEN PREVIOUS SURGERY?	• *Post gastrectomy* (dumping syndrome): small, frequent snacks. If severe, consider octreotide. • *Intestinal resection* (causing bile salt irritation of colon): cholestyramine 12-16G daily + ranitidine. • *Blind loop* (causing bacterial overgrowth): tetracycline (or metronidazole) for 2-4 weeks. • *Blind rectum with ostomy* (causing mucus discharge) - see notes on p60.

Clinical decision	If YES → Action
IS STOOL MIXED WITH BLOOD OR DISCHARGE?	• *Fungating rectal or colonic tumour:* topical corticosteroids (prednisolone enema) ± metronidazole 500mg 12-hourly. Use topical sucralfate or tranexamic acid to control bleeding close to anal margin. Consider radiotherapy. • *Infection* (eg. shigella, salmonella, clostridium): identify and treat. • *Inflammation:* assess cause and treat.
IS CLEAR FLUID PRESENT IN THE STOOL?	**If volume less than 1 litre per 24 hours:** • *Mucus* (total bowel obstruction / blind rectum / rectal or colonic tumour secreting mucus): hyoscine butylbromide may help (SC infusion 60-300 mg per 24 hours). • *Urine* (vesicocolic or vesicorectal fistula): catheter or desmopressin at night (see **Urinary problems**). **Volume more than 1 litre per 24 hours** (usually secretory): • *Infective:* avoid loperamide or atropine. Rehydration as opposite. If persistent: stool microscopy and microbiology and treat on the advice of a microbiologist. • *Tumour secreting vasoactive intestinal peptide (VIPoma):* octreotide (see below). • *Carcinoid:* start ranitidine or omeprazole. Consider octreotide (see below).
IS DIARRHOEA PERSISTING?	• Exclude: *Drugs:* excess laxatives, antibiotics, NSAID's, b-blockers, diuretics, Mg++ antacids *Infection:* send 3 stool specimens (in AIDS up to 6 stool specimens may be needed, and for CMV or adenovirus a rectal biopsy may be required). *Gastrocolic or enterorectal fistula:* consider colostomy. *Irritable colon:* increase dietary fibre. *Anxiety, fear:* see **The anxious person**. *Faecal incontinence due to neurological or sphincter dysfunction:* consider a colostomy. If time is available, start a bowel management programme.[200] *Autonomic insufficiency:* clonidine may help in diabetes. • Treat symptomatically: Loperamide 2-4mg with each loose stool (up to 32mg daily may be needed in AIDS related diarrhoea). Stop laxatives and Mg++ antacids. Consider: hyoscine butylbromide SC infusion 60-300 mg per 24 hours **or** octreotide SC infusion 150 - 300 microg. per 24 hrs. Protective ointment or hydrocolloid dressings to perineum and anal margin. Consider perineal stool collecting bag if stool volume is large.

Adapted from Regnard and Mannix [198]

NOTES

Rehydration: simple oral rehydration powders are available (eg. Dioralyte). The WHO rehydration formula is an alternative (for each litre of water: 3.5g NaCl, 2.5g $NaHCO_3$, 1.5g KCl and 20g glucose or 40g sucrose)[199]. Any powder must have exactly the recommended amount of water added- too much will reduce the efficacy, too little risks hypernatraemia. Parenteral rehydration is used if the fluid loss is severe and Ringer lactate solution is preferred.[199]

Blood loss into the upper gastrointestinal tract irritates the bowel producing a loose, dark or black stool. Blood loss from the small bowel or colon may be reduced with systemic tranexamic acid. Bleeding from a rectal tumour will lessen with topical sucralfate[162] or topical tranexamic acid.[164]

Steatorrhoea is due to excessive fat in the stool. Ranitidine will increase fat absorption since this makes duodenal contents less acid and encourages lipid micelle formation that is an essential step to lipid absorption in the small bowel. This is particularly important in pancreatic insufficiency (where alkaline pancreatic secretions are reduced), and following small bowel resection (where gastric acid output increases due to raised gastrin). Omeprazole is a more potent gastric acid inhibitor and is often necessary in Zollinger Ellison syndrome.

Previous surgery can cause diarrhoea through a number of mechanisms. Gastrectomy patients can suffer from food being 'dumped' into the bowel causing nausea, bloating and diarrhoea. If bile salts escape into the colon they cause local irritation and this may occur because ileal resection has prevented their reabsorption.

Loperamide increases water absorption by slowing forward peristalsis. Caution is necessary with infective diarrhoea since this action can cause overgrowth of dangerous pathogens and increased absorption of bacterial toxins.

Post-radiotherapy diarrhoea can respond to nonsteroidal anti-inflammatory drugs.[201, 202] If pelvic radiotherapy causes a proctitis, adjust laxatives to keep the stool soft.

Octreotide has been used in AIDS-related diarrhoea,[203] in postgrastectomy dumping, and may also have a role to play in other causes of severe refractory diarrhoea,[204] (100 micrograms SC 8-hourly, or 300 micrograms SC infusion per 24hrs).

Diabetes in advanced disease

Clinical decision	If YES → Action
IS TREATMENT URGENT?	see **Emergencies:** Diabetes
IS PATIENT SYMPTOMATIC?	• *Hypoglycaemia:* reduce dose of insulin or oral hypoglycaemics. It is common to be able to stop these as the illness progresses. Exclude other causes of hypoglycaemia (adrenocortical insufficiency, insulinomas, non-selective ß-blockers, pentamidine, post gastrectomy dumping) and treat appropriately. • *Hyperglycaemia:* Exclude drug causes of hyperglycaemia (corticosteroids, octreotide, diuretics). If drug is essential, start an oral hypoglycaemic agent. *If previously a diabetic:* titrate insulin or oral hypoglycaemic agent. Once daily insulin regimens are usually possible (eg. Ultratard).[207]
WAS PATIENT PREVIOUSLY DIABETIC?	• Expect to reduce doses of insulin and hypoglycaemics as illness progresses. • Maintain blood glucose in whatever range avoids symptoms (usually 8-15mmol/l) (tight control to prevent future complications is not appropriate).

NOTES

Causes of hypoglycaemia: this is most commonly due to reducing requirements for insulin or oral hypoglycaemic agents as the illness progresses. Unusual causes are adrenocortical insufficiency, insulinomas, non-selective b-blockers, pentamidine and post gastrectomy dumping.

Causes of hyperglycaemia: some patients developed diabetes prior to their current illness, such as insulin dependent diabetes (IDDM types Ia and Ib), non-insulin dependent diabetes (NIDDM type II, obese or non-obese) or malnutrition-related diabetes (type III). Secondary causes include pancreatic disease (pancreatitis, occasionally pancreatic carcinoma), drugs (corticosteroids, octreotide, diuretics), hormone producing tumours (glugagonomas, phaeochromocytoma) and various genetic syndromes (glycogen storage disease, Huntingdon's chorea, Laurence-Moon-Biedl, Werner's).[205] In addition, cancer patients have increased gluconeogenesis, reduced glucose tolerance and increased insulin resistance.[206]

Managing hyperglycaemia: the aim is to minimise symptoms, not the tight control of blood glucose.[207] Glucose ranges of 8-15 mmol are acceptable as long as patients are asymptomatic. Patients who have a history of hyperglycaemia may tolerate higher levels, and may develop hypoglycaemic symptoms at levels of 2-6mmol/l. Drowsiness, confusion or coma require urgent treatment. In hyperglycaemia the main goals are to rehydrate, restore a normal BP, treat hypoxia, and reduce glucose while maintaining potassium levels. Both ketotic and non-ketotic hyperglycaemia can be treated in this way. Ketotic patients will be acidotic, and it is appropriate to treat this with bicarbonate if they are hyperventilating, but in patients with advanced disease closer control is best done where blood gases can be easily monitored.

Physical symptoms:
NOTES AND REVISIONS (regular revision updates available on CLIP Update Service)

Physical symptoms:
NOTES AND REVISIONS (regular revision updates available on CLIP Update Service)

Psychological symptoms

Communications, like tumours, may be benign or malignant. They may also be invasive, and the effects of bad communication with a patient may metastasise to the family.
Michael Simpson
Professor of Psychiatry and Family Medicine [1]

Confusional states

Clinical decision	If YES→Action

- Provide company, a constant routine and a light, quiet environment.
- Always assume a patient understands.

IS MEMORY FAILURE PRESENT?	**If there is a previous history suggesting dementia** (failure to retain information, little fluctuation in confusion, no change in alertness): • Orientate frequently in time, place and person. • Ensure constant environment, encourage activity. • *If cerebral tumour is present:* start high dose dexamethasone and consider cranial irradiation.
HAS ALERTNESS CHANGED?	• *If dehydrated:* see **Reduced hydration and feeding**. • Consider drugs (many drugs can cause confusion- check current datasheet). Stop all except absolutely essential drugs. Reduce dose of essential drugs or change to alternatives. • Consider drug or alcohol withdrawal: restart drug or alcohol. • Exclude infection: reduce pyrexia, examine chest, test urine. Treat as appropriate • Exclude biochemical cause: (hypercalcaemia, uraemia, inappropriate ADH secretion) - treat if possible and appropriate. • Exclude cardiac or respiratory disease: (ventricular failure, pleural effusion, pulmonary metastases) - treat if possible and appropriate. • Exclude recent trauma: (long bone fracture, subdural haematoma).
IS CONCENTRATION IMPAIRED?	**In presence of anxiety:** • Consider: ignorance about diagnosis, communication problems, social problems. **In absence of anxiety:** • Consider: distraction due to pain, psychiatric illness (eg. anxiety state, depression).
IS PATIENT EXPERIENCING UNUSUAL SIGHTS OR SOUNDS?	**If seeing or hearing things:** • Ensure a light, quiet and consistent environment. • *If patient is misinterpreting an external stimulus:* - review causes of altered alertness above. • *If patient is hallucinating (no external stimulus):* -exclude drugs, or chemical withdrawal. -control with haloperidol or levomepromazine (methotrimeprazine) - see opposite. -consider a psychotic illness and refer as appropriate.
HAS BEHAVIOUR ALTERED?	**If patient is wandering, paranoid, euphoric, manic or depressive:** • Exclude causes of memory failure as above. • Consider drugs (especially corticosteroids). • Consider psychiatric illness and refer as appropriate.

- **Explain** cause of confusion, possible treatment and management to patient (and to family and staff).

Adapted from Stedeford and Regnard [2]

Clinical decision	If YES → Action
IS CONTROL OF DISTURBANCE URGENT?	Use the following for emergency treatment while awaiting assessment or treatment: • Ensure well-lit, quiet, constant environment. **In absence of abnormal experience or behaviour:** Use benzodiazepine: • *For minimal sedation:* lorazepam 0.5-1mg PO or sublingually. • *If sedation required:* midazolam 2-10mg SC, IM or PR 1-hourly as required (or 20-120mg SC infusion per 24 hours). **In the presence of abnormal experience or behaviour:** Use antipsychotic: • *For minimal sedation:* haloperidol 2.5-10mg once at night PO or SC. • *If sedation required:* thioridazine 25-50mg PO at night **or** levomepromazine (methotrimeprazine) 12.5-100mg 8-hourly PO or SC or as SC infusion 25-300mg per 24 hours). **If disturbance persists:** Use combination of benzodiazepine and antipsychotic.

Adapted from Stedeford and Regnard [2]

NOTES

Acute and chronic confusional states: *acute confusional states* are the commonest form of confusion in advanced disease. It is present if there are 4 or more features[3]. Six are highly specific: acute onset, fluctuating course, disorganised thinking, inattention, memory impairment, and disorientation. Five are less specific: altered sleep-awake cycle, abnormal psychomotor activity, altered level of consciousness, and perceptual disturbance. *Chronic confusional states* are seen in the dementias. They can have similar features to acute states, but the history is longer, the symptoms fluctuate less, and the patient's alertness is unlikely to have changed.

Memory failure: this is common in confusional states and is usually due to a reversible failure to take in information. In the dementias there is a failure to retain information because of irreversible cortical damage.

Alteration in alertness: this can be either an increase or decrease in alertness. In the dementias, alertness is unchanged. Drugs and infection are the commonest causes. Hypercalcaemia should always be suspected in patients with malignancy who have unexplained confusion.

Impaired concentration: this can occur independently of any change in alertness. An extreme form is seen in 'frozen terror' where severe anxiety produces a state of immobile withdrawal.[4]

Abnormal experiences: misperceptions and hallucinations need to be differentiated.[5] *Misperceptions* have an external stimulus and occur with reduced alertness or concentration. A patient may think they see someone to one side, only to turn and find no-one is there. *Hallucinations* are much less common, have no outside stimulus and appear real. This differentiation is important with morphine since misperceptions will usually disappear as tolerance to drowsiness occurs, whereas hallucinations require a change in dose or opioid.

Altered behaviour: this can cause the most difficulties in managing a confused patient. When due to a reversible, acute confusional state, treating the cause of the confusion will return the behaviour to normal.

Explanation: confusional states can be frightening for all involved: the patients fear they are 'losing their mind' while carers feel uneasy at the unpredictability of the patient's words and actions. Confused patients can understand explanations, although if their concentration is impaired this explanation may have to be repeated several times.

Urgent control of disturbance: occasionally the behaviour risks harm to the patients or others. Because escape and paranoia are two common features it may take a great deal of explanation and a calm, well-lit environment. If medication is unavoidable, it is best to start with drugs with minimal sedation unless the disturbance is severe. In the absence of abnormal behaviour, anxiety and fear are prominent and benzodiazepines will help suppress the anxiety to a level that is manageable for the patient. When abnormal behaviour is present, antipsychotic medication is needed, although a few patients need both.

The anxious person

The initial approach

Clinical decision	If YES → Action

DOES PERSON FEEL VERY APPREHENSIVE, TENSE OR ON EDGE?	• Exclude drug-induced motor restlessness- dyskinesia (patient appears restless but may deny any anxiety) (see notes for list of drugs): Stop drug.
	• Start supportive measures:
	    Supportive communication
	    Offer information if patient wishes this (if information is likely to be difficult news see **Breaking difficult news**).
	    Explore causes of anxiety by encouragement to disclose concerns (see **Eliciting current problems**).
	    Look for links between thoughts and feelings.
	    Explore possible solutions eg. by helping the person to reframe more realistic interpretations or visualise more positive images.
	    Review procedures causing anxiety.

CAN AN ANXIETY STATE BE EXCLUDED?	**If this is moderate anxiety:** • Teach relaxation exercises (distraction, autogenic relaxation). • Enable access to aromatherapy and massage.

IS AN ANXIETY STATE PRESENT?	Characteristics:
	    Persistent apprehension (> 2 weeks and for >50% of time).
	    This is different to their usual mood.
	    Four or more features of anxiety are present (see notes)
	• Go to clinical decisions on opposite page.

Adapted from Maguire, Faulkner and Regnard [6]

NOTES

Anxiety: life-threatening illness creates an uncertain future that causes anxiety which may increase as the illness progresses. Anxiety in turn makes it more difficult for the patient to cope with suffering. Features of anxiety are *apprehensive expectation* (eg. fear, rumination, tendency to perceive situations in a threatening way), *vigilance and scanning* (eg. irritability, poor concentration, difficulty getting to sleep, tendency to perceive bodily sensations in a threatening way), *motor tension* (eg. trembling, tension, restlessness) and *autonomic hyperactivity* (eg. sweating, dry mouth, cold hands, tachycardia, diarrhoea). In advanced disease, anxiety is often associated with depression. The Hospital Anxiety and Depression (HAD) scale is a sensitive and specific tool for generalised anxiety.[7, 12]

Drug induced restlessness (dyskinesia): this is unrelated to anxiety but can mimic the motor tension aspects of anxiety. Drugs which may cause this are cyclizine, haloperidol, hyoscine, levomepromazine (methotrimeprazine), metoclopramide, and the tricyclic antidepressants (eg. amitriptyline). The differentiating feature is that patients may deny any severe anxiety. Occasionally drug induced motor restlessness co-exists with anxiety, and the only way to uncover its existence is to try a trial without the incriminating drugs. A single drug alone is an unusual cause unless high doses are being used, or the patients is very young or elderly. The risk is much greater when two or more at-risk drugs are used together and this risk can be reduced by avoiding combinations of drugs with this effect.

Supportive measures: enabling a person to express their feelings and giving the information they need can do much to ease anxiety. Helping the individual to look for links between thoughts and feelings can generate more realistic interpretations. For example, feeling 'out of control with all that machinery.' can be changed into, 'It's good to think all that technology is there to help.' Similar approaches have been used with visualisation. Anxiety management techniques can be helpful such as distraction or relaxation. Muscle relaxation techniques are best avoided as it can worsen the anxiety of some people who are excessively vigilant of their bodily sensations and autogenic relaxation is a better alternative. There should also be access to other help with relaxation such as massage or aromatherapy. Reflexology has a role if the therapist is willing to pass any interpretations they make to the professional and not to the patient (telling an anxious person the reflexologist 'felt something wrong' with their kidney will worsen their anxiety).

Helping the person with an anxiety state

Clinical decision	If YES→Action
IS PERSON FUNCTIONING POORLY?	**If disorganisation is severe** (tormented, unable to care for self or make a decision): • Start antipsychotic: *For minimal sedation:* use haloperidol 5-20mg at night. *If sedation is needed:* use levomepromazine (methotrimeprazine)25-50mg 8-hourly PO or SC. **If disorganisation is moderate** (poor concentration, but is caring for self): • Start benzodiazepine: *For minimal sedation:* lorazepam 0.5-1mg PO or sublingually. *If sedation required:* temazepam 10-20mg 8-hourly. **If disorganisation persists:** • Refer for specialist help and advice.
ARE SOMATIC SYMPTOMS PROMINENT?	ie. autonomic hyperactivity (eg. tremor, tachycardia, sweating, diarrhoea). • Consider a β-blocker eg. propranaolol 10-40mg 8-hourly (NB. risk of hypotension if used with lorazepam, temazepam or levomepromazine).
DO SUDDEN PANICS OR PHOBIC EPISODES OCCUR?	• Seek out triggers and explore thoughts. • Consider clomipramine 25mg at night (10mg if >70 years). • Consider referral for cognitive therapy if available.

• **Start supportive measures** (see opposite).

IS THE SITUATION PERSISTING?	Patient remains very apprehensive, tense, or on edge. • Consider the concurrent presence of depression (see **The withdrawn patient**). • Refer for specialist advice and help.

Adapted from Maguire, Faulkner and Regnard [6]

Anxiety state: this has an dominating and intrusive quality- even normally anxious people will describe a significant increase in the intensity and frequency of their anxiety. Unlike other times of anxiety, they will find themselves unable to pull out of this by themselves. An anxiety state therefore represents a change in mood, is persistent, dominating and accompanied by at least four anxiety-related symptoms (see opposite). Some of these symptoms may be due to the underlying disease process (eg. impaired concentration, fatigue).

Disorganised functioning: as anxiety worsens the individual becomes increasingly distracted from daily activities. As it becomes more severe it begins to intrude on everyday decisions such as what to wear, or whether to get washed. Decisions become increasingly made on the spur of the moment and erratic. Moderate disorganisation will ease with anxiety suppressants such as the benzodiazepines, but severe disorganisation will require antipsychotics.

Panic: these occur suddenly without an obvious cause, are intense and can last 5-20 minutes. A fear of dying and loss of control are often provoked by the episodes. Although there is no obvious warning, individuals can be taught to identify triggers or specific thoughts that precede a panic. These thoughts may give some clue as the cause, but also provide a means of instituting self-taught controls that with practice can prevent thoughts of panic developing into full episode.

Phobias: situations or objects are interpreted as occasions when help is impossible, difficult or embarrassing. If individuals feel humiliated by these feelings they will find it hard to disclose their phobia. Treatment is similar to panic disorders.

Specialist support: help will be needed to unravel mixed disorders (eg. mixed anxiety and depression), to diagnose unusual presentations, deal with a persistent anxiety state or provide further counselling.[4, 14] This help may be from a psychiatrist, psychologist, counsellor or social worker. In reality it is more likely to depend on what is available locally.

The withdrawn patient

Helping the withdrawn patient

Clinical decision	If YES → Action
IS THIS USUAL BEHAVIOUR?	Normally introverted or quiet personality • Offer time to establish trust.

• **Establish dialogue:** acknowledge difficulties (eg. 'It's clear we're having difficulty getting into a conversation.') and negotiate further discussion (eg. 'Can you bear to tell me why you find it so difficult to talk to me just now?').

Clinical decision	If YES → Action
IS PATIENT UNWILLING TO CONTINUE?	• Acknowledge the patient's refusal to continue. • Offer willingness to help in the future if needed.
IS THERE A CONFUSIONAL STATE ?	See **Confusional states**.
COULD THERE BE AN ORGANIC CAUSE?	• Exclude drugs causing parkinsonism (eg. haloperidol, metoclopramide, levomepromazine). • Consider parkinsonism due to brain damage (eg. encephalitis, dementia, tumour). • Fatigue and weakness related to the illness: see **Fatigue and weakness**.
IS ANGER PRESENT?	• See **The angry person**.
ARE FEARS, GUILT OR SHAME PRESENT?	• Identify, clarify and specify concerns (see **Eliciting current problems**). • *If patient is apprehensive, tense or on edge:* see **The anxious person**. • *If guilt or shame are present:* If this is realistic check if patient could accept self-forgiveness. If this is unrealistic help a patient to reframe thoughts about the emotion.
IS PATIENT APATHETIC, OR FEELING HELPLESS?	**If a depressive illness is present** Persistent low mood (>4 weeks for >50% of time) This is different to their usual mood. Difficult or impossible to distract out of low mood Four other depressive-related symptoms (see notes). • Commence supportive counselling • Start lofepramine 70mg at night (titrating up to 280mg daily in divided doses).
IS CONDITION PERSISTING?	• Refer for specialist advice and help.

Adapted from Maguire, Faulkner and Regnard [8]

NOTES

Withdrawal: this has many possible causes and these should be excluded before assuming a depression is present. A drug-induced parkinsonism, for example, will reduce a patient's facial expressions (which may be interpreted as a low mood) and mobility (which may be interpreted as motor retardation due to depression). Even a normal, introverted, quiet personality can seem depressed without careful enquiry.

Depression: one quarter of cancer and AIDS patients suffer from depression.[9] It is therefore important to screen for depression in patients with advanced disease. The Hospital Anxiety and Depression (HAD) scale is not sensitive or specific enough for depression, and the Brief Assessment Schedule Cards may be better suited for this population.[7, 10] Netherthless, the HAD scale can help detect unsuspected or probable cases and provides a simple means of monitoring improvement. The key features of a depression are a change of mood, a pervasive and persistent low mood, a difficulty to be easily distracted out of that low mood, and four or more depressive symptoms. These symptoms may include a diurnal variation in mood, repeated or early morning wakening, impaired concentration, loss of interest or enjoyment, and feelings of hopelessness, guilt, shame or feeling a burden to others. In advanced disease antidepressants are still the quickest way to achieve a response and if the depression started recently, the response may occur in under 3 weeks. Lofepramine is the antidepressant of choice, with the best balance of efficacy and adverse effects, but cognitive therapy is also helpful.[11] If the depression persists it is essential to ask for advice and help from psychiatry colleagues.[14]

The angry person

Clinical decision	If YES → Action

- **Acknowledge what anger does to you** (if such situations always make you very angry or very passive, ask someone else to conduct the interview).

IS THE PERSON CONTROLLED AND CONTAINED?	• Check whether the anger is solely with you or another carer. If it is, the angry carer should withdraw and seek support. **If this is passive anger:** • Acknowledge the anger (eg. 'Am I right that this has made you angry?'). • Negotiate to discuss cause (eg. 'Can you explain why you're feeling like this?') • Encourage the expression of anger (eg. 'Just how angry have you been?'). • Avoid the temptation to defend yourself or others.
IS THE ANGER APPROPRIATE?	**If the anger is misdirected** (eg. anger at a GP that chemotherapy failed): • Check this (eg. 'I can see that you're angry that the treatment didn't work, but could you tell me why your anger is directed at me?'). • Explore the causes of anger that may be uncovered. **If the anger is correctly directed** (eg. appointments are running 1 hour late): • Identify the level of anger. • Show understanding without being defensive (eg. 'I'd be angry too.'). • Enable them to express their anger. • Apologise if you have made an error (do not apologise for others).
IS THE ANGER ESCALATING?	• Position yourself near room exit with door open. • Set limits (eg. 'I can see you're finding it hard to control your anger, but I can only continue if you feel you can keep in control. Can you do that?') **If person cannot accept limits = pathological anger** • **Stop the interview and leave the room immediately.** (eg. 'In that case I have to stop this discussion now.')
IS THE PERSON DEPRESSED?	eg. apathetic or expressing feelings of hopelessness. • See **The withdrawn patient**.
IS THE ANGER CAUSING ISOLATION?	• Acknowledge their isolation (eg. 'Your anger seems to have left you lonely.') • Explore the effects of the isolation on relationships.
IS THE ANGER PERSISTING?	• Is this normal behaviour? • Are there causes unconnected to the illness? • Ask for specialist advice and help for the person (eg. cognitive therapy).

Adapted from Faulkner, Maguire and Regnard [13]

NOTES

Anger: advanced illness produces many reasons to be angry such as unrealised ambitions, loss of control, feelings of hopelessness, depression, and spiritual conflicts. This may be expressed passively (controlled anger) or actively. The anger may be appropriate to the situation or be out of proportion. Finally it may correctly directed or misdirected. Anger that is actively expressed, appropriate and correctly directed is easier to help than anger that is passive, out of proportion or misdirected. No assumptions should be made about the anger until it has been assessed.

Pathological anger: angry people are asking to be heard. If this opportunity is given by acknowledging the anger and listening to its reasons, most people's anger will start to defuse. In a few people the opposite happens. This warning sign must be heeded since there is a risk that it will be followed by violence.

Persisting anger: some people have always reacted angrily to situations and they or their partners will admit to this. Others have reasons for their anger that are unrelated to the illness. Occasionally anger is part of other conditions such as depression and the advice and help of a specialist can be invaluable.[4, 14]

Psychological symptoms:
NOTES AND REVISIONS (regular revision updates available on CLIP update service)

Psychological symptoms:
NOTES AND REVISIONS (regular revision updates available on CLIP update service)

Emergencies

If the deterioration is unexpected: start with clinical decisions on unexpected deterioration.

Dealing with emergencies:
The aim is to consider each stage within the time suggested, while planning the next step.
In this way urgent situations become a series of achievable goals, so reducing fear for both patient and carer.

Emergencies

Unexpected deterioration: making decisions

Clinical decision	If YES →Action
ARE DRUGS THE CAUSE?	• Reduce dose. **If ventilation has been seriously compromised** (<5 resps / min): *Opioids:* dilute 1mg naloxone in 10mls 0.9% saline and titrate IV at 0.1mg/min. until respiration improves, followed by naloxone infusion. *Spinal anaesthetics:* IV fluids, 3-9mg ephedrine IV if hypotensive, ventilation may be needed for 1-2 hours. *Benzodiazepine:* flumazenil IV 200microg. over 15 seconds followed by 100microg / minute up to 1000microg (1mg).
IS TREATMENT INDICATED FOR COMFORT ONLY?	eg. rapid deterioration with irreversible cause (eg. massive haemoptysis, haematemesis or pulmonary embolus), very short prognosis (hour by hour deterioration), or patient refusing treatment • Sedation if agitated (see **Emergencies:** agitation) • Analgesia if in pain (see **Emergencies:** severe pain) • Support of patient, partner, family and staff (including you!).
IS TREATMENT OF THE CAUSE CLEARLY APPROPRIATE?	• Arrange necessary investigations and treat the cause of deterioration • *If there is to be a delay in treatment and patient is distressed:* give sedation (see **Emergencies:** agitation).
IS THE NEED FOR TREATMENT UNCERTAIN?	• Consult with the partner or family as they may offer useful information (eg. previously stated refusal to treatment). • Consult with the care team taking into account history, rate of deterioration, availability of treatment and previous quality of life. **If need is still unclear use the rule of 3:** Hour by hour deterioration: review in 3 hours. Day by day deterioration: review in 3 days. • *If further deterioration has occurred:* treat for comfort. • *If no further deterioration:* consider treating.

Notes

In the presence of advanced, irreversible disease additional factors can cause unexpected deterioration (eg. hypercalcaemia). It is usually clear whether treatment is appropriate or not, but the complexity of the situation can make such decisions difficult.

Drugs can mimic deterioration due to the disease. If the deterioration is unexpected (ie. the drug was not given with the intention to sedate), then the dose should be reduced. Patients have the right to be as alert and aware as possible if this is their wish.

Comfort only required: the deterioration may be unequivocally irreversible (eg. massive haemoptysis), or the patient may have already been deteriorating rapidly because of their primary condition. Alternatively, the patient (or the partner on the patient's behalf) may unequivocally refuse further treatment. In these situations the treatment is aimed at relieving distress and achieving comfort.

Is the need still uncertain? Even after taking all the details into consideration, including discussion with the patient and partner or family, on occasions it can still be difficult to know how appropriate it is to treat the cause of the deterioration. Waiting a short time will often resolve the situation. If the situation remains unchanged this suggests the patient has sufficient reserves to undergo treatment of the primary cause, while continuing deterioration suggests treatment should be for comfort only.

Severe pain

Clinical decision	If YES → Action
Immediately **IS PAIN CONTROL** **URGENT?**	**Achieve sufficient comfort to allow initial assessment.** • Find comfortable position (padding/splint). • Give diamorphine SC, IM or IV (5mg if not on opioid, otherwise use equivalent of usual 4-hourly dose). • *For agitation:* see **Emergencies:** severe agitation • *For colic:* hyoscine butylbromide 20mg SC, IM or IV • *For a myocardial infarction:* treat as appropriate. NB. Choice of route: SC is kindest but slowest, use IM or IV if rapid response needed (minimum wait for reassessment after SC = 30mins; after IM = 20mins; after IV= 2mins)
Within 1 hour **IS THE PAIN WORSENED** **BY THE SLIGHTEST** **PASSIVE MOVEMENT?**	**Exclude causes requiring urgent management.** • *For back pain:* exclude cord compression- see **Emergencies:** spinal cord compression • *If pathological fracture suspected:* decide if the patient is able to travel for an X-ray.
Within 4 hours **IS PAIN PRESENT AT** **REST?**	**Achieve comfort at rest** • *If still in pain at rest:* if not on an opioid, start morphine. Otherwise increase regular opioid dose by 50%. Consider contacting pain or palliative care specialist. • *If several opioid dose increases have been ineffective:* try ketamine SC infusion 50-100mg per 24 hours (see **Drug formulary** for details). • *If still in pain at rest and further treatment is to be delayed for more than 6 hours:* consider light sedation with SC infusion of midazolam 30mg per 24 hours plus diamorphine at equivalent of current dose (see p19 for equivalent doses).
Within 24 hours **IS PAIN CONTROL** **NEEDED FOR MORE** **THAN 5 DAYS?**	**Plan for stable pain control** • Check through the clinical decisions 2-10 starting on p13. • Ensure a good night's sleep using sedatives if necessary. • If pain is localised (eg. fracture), consider ketamine or spinal analgesia. **Within 1 week:** plan for managing any psychological consequences. See sections on **Anxiety**, **Anger**, **Withdrawal** (the presence of these problems may delay resolution of the pain for several weeks).

NOTES

Severe pain: the most immediate goal is to reduce pain at rest and to allow the patient to settle sufficiently to allow adequate assessment. Agitation driven by fear and pain will ease with titrated midazolam- some patients will require no more than 2.5mg (eg. ill patients or those who have slept little in the previous 24 hours), others will require more than 10mg (eg. younger patients or those previously on benzodiazepines). Simple treatments for some pathological fractures are possible eg. splinting for a humeral neck fracture, or intercostal nerve block for a rib fracture. An intercostal block of bupivacaine and methylprednisolone (as DepoMedrone) gives analgesia for as long as radiotherapy.[1] Other fractures (eg. vertebra, femoral shaft) will need ketamine, local nerve blocks or spinal analgesia. In situations when a procedure is to be delayed (eg. in the night), or where a patient is deteriorating rapidly, titrated sedation is appropriate. The advice of palliative care, pain and oncology colleagues can be invaluable. Although the agitation may settle, low mood, anxiety and exhaustion may persist (see **the Anxious Person**, **the Angry Person**, **the Withdrawn patient**). This persistence of psychological problems will delay the resolution of the pain for several weeks and to avoid disappointment this needs to be understood by patient, partner and staff.[2]

Severe agitation

Clinical decision	If YES → Action
Immediately **IS CONTROL OF AGITATION URGENT?**	**eg. irreversible haemorrhage, prevention of injury to patient:** • Midazolam 2-10mg titrated IV, **or** 5mg IM / PR repeated as necessary intil the patient is settled. • Ensure environment is safe (eg. placing mattress on floor). • Massage **may** help. • Do not leave patient unattended. • Do not use opiods to treat the agitation. • *If hypoxic:* commence oxygen (100% through face mask, 24% if previous pulmonary disease with carbon dioxide retention). and see **Respiratory problems**.
Within 1 hour **IS THERE EVIDENCE OF ABNORMAL EXPERIENCE OR BEHAVIOUR?**	**Reduce agitation sufficiently to enable assessment:** eg. hallucinations, paranoia (see also p64). • Haloperidol: 5-10mg IM, repeated SC hourly (up to maximum of 50mg) until agitation lessens while avoiding sedation if possible. • Do not leave patient unattended. • *If fear is the only feature:* for minimal sedation use lorazepam 0.5 - 1mg sublingually or orally. For sedation: midazolam 2.5 - 5mg SC/PR, repeated SC hourly if necessary.
Within 4 hours **IS AGITATION STILL PRESENT?**	**Plan for control of agitation:** • *With minimal sedation:* -if abnormal experiences or behaviour: haloperidol 5-20mg SC infusion/24hrs. -with fear as only feature: lorazepam 0.5-2mg SL 8-hourly. • *With sedation:* -if abnormal experiences or behaviour: levomepromazine (methotrimeprazine) 25-300mg SC infusion/24 hours. -with fear as only feature: midazolam 20-120mg SC infusion/ 24 hours. • *If agitation persists:* phenobarbital SC infusion 800-1600mg per 24 hours.[3] Do not use opioids to treat the agitation.
Within 24 hours **CAN CAUSE BE TREATED?**	**Assess cause of agitation:** • Exclude causes of confusional states (see **Confusional states**). • Exclude factors that exacerbate a confusional state (eg. full rectum, urinary retention, pain, discomfort). • Exclude fear.

NOTES

Severe agitation: the aims are to reduce the agitation sufficiently for comfort, and to find a treatable cause if possible. Sedation should be kept to a minimum since it will make it difficult for the patient to understand what is happening and will hinder assessment. Sedation may be necessary when the cause is irreversible (eg. renal failure due to ureters obstructed by tumour), or when a patient is deteriorating rapidly (day by day). Ideally, sedation needs the permission of the patient, but this is not usually possible to obtain in severe agitation. In this situation it is important to have agreement from the partner or relative.

Opiods are contraindicated as a treatment of agitation since they make the agitation worse through the accumulation of active metabolites, and tolerance to the sedating effect ocurs rapidly.

Hypercalcaemia in advanced cancer

Clinical decision	If YES → Action
Immediately **IS HYPERCALCAEMIA PRESENT?**	**Assess and treat symptoms:** (Suspect hypercalcaemia if unexplained nausea, vomiting, drowsiness, confusion, constipation, thirst or polyuria) • Treat symptoms of hypercalcaemia: see **Constipation**, **Nausea and vomiting**, and **Confusional states**.
Within 24 hours **IS TREATMENT APPROPRIATE?**	**Confirm diagnosis and commence treatment:** • Take blood for serum calcium **and** albumin, or ionised calcium. • If hypercalcaemic (corrected serum Ca^{++}>2.8) give 60-90mg pamidronate as 4-hour IV infusion in 500mls 0.9% saline. **If dehydrated:** • Arrange for 72 hours IV hydration. **If patient is too agitated for IV pamidronate:** • See **Emergencies**: severe agitation. **If hydration good:** • Ensure oral hydration of at least 1.5 litres/24 hours.
Over next month **HAS HYPERCALCAEMIA RECURRED?**	**Delay recurrence, treat recurrences early:** • Recheck calcium at first sign of symptoms returning. -if raised give pamidronate as single infusion (can be done as outpatient or at home). • Review antitumour therapy.

NOTES

Hypercalcaemia is common in some cancers (50% of myeloma, 25% of bronchial carcinomas and 20% of breast carcinomas).[4,5] In 80% of cases the cause is the production of a parathyroid hormone-related protein by the tumour,[5,6] a process which is unrelated to the presence of bone metastases. Symptoms are insidious and mimic deterioration due to cancer. Drowsiness, nausea, vomiting, confusion, constipation or thirst may occur, but often as a single symptom. Polyuria is also usual, but is very difficult to detect from history alone. Patients who were well 1-2 weeks previously and unexpectedly seem to have deteriorated may be hypercalcaemic. Such patients should have blood taken for biochemistry: ionised calcium or serum calcium plus albumin- in the latter case the calcium must be corrected for a low albumin:[7] true serum Ca^{++} = [(40 - albumin) x 0.025] + serum calcium. Values of serum calcium >2.8 mmol/l are abnormal.

Steroids are only effective in myeloma and lymphoma.[5] For all other tumours the bisphosphonates are now the most effective treatment available. Pamidronate is given as a single 2 or 4 hour infusion of 60-90mg. Since dehydration can be profound due to the polyuria, 72 hours of IV hydration is often necessary, but will not by itself achieve useful control of the hypercalcaemia.[5,8] There is a 48 hour delay before the pamidronate begins to act and therefore it is our practice to give pamidronate at the outset of treatment, particularly as effective rehydration will help to reduce the calcium in the first 72 hours. Frusemide IV has been used to further lower calcium levels, but the benefit is unclear and it may cause additional electrolyte disturbances.[5] Following pamidronate, retreatment may be needed in 2-4 weeks,[9] but the patient is now alert to the symptoms and treatment can begin before the calcium level is high, and a single 2 hour infusion as an outpatient or at home is often all that is necessary. Oral bisphosphonates delay, rather than prevent, the need for an infusion. Most patients return to their pre-hypercalcaemic state with a good quality of life. Hypercalcaemia is an indicator of disease progression, however, and breast cancer patients in particular may require a change in their hormone treatment.

Superior vena caval obstruction (SVCO) in advanced cancer

Clinical decision	If YES → Action
Immediately **IS SVCO PRESENT?**	**Confirm SVCO:** • Consider SVCO if there is: oedema of face or arms, distended neck and arm veins, headache, dusky colour to skin in chest, arms and face. **Commence urgent treatment:** • Give dexamethasone 24mg IV as slow injection over 2 minutes. • If stridor present: see table below. • Start dexamethasone 18mg PO in divided doses.
IS TREATMENT **APPROPRIATE?**	**Arrange definitive treatment:** • Contact clinical oncologist to consider urgent X-ray and radiotherapy, chemotherapy or SVC stent • Continue high dose dexamethasone until after radiotherapy and reduce to lowest dose that controls symptoms.

Stridor in advanced cancer

Clinical decision	If YES → Action
Immediately **IS STRIDOR PRESENT?**	**Confirm stridor:** • Consider if there is rasping sound or wheeze from upper airway. **Commence urgent treatment:** • If patient is very agitated: see **Emergencies:** severe agitation • If available: start 4:1 helium/oxygen mixture. • Give dexamethasone 24mg IV as slow injection over 2 minutes. • Explanation, air movement, sitting upright, and massage can help. • Continue dexamethasone 18mg daily.
IS VOICE HOARSE OR **WHISPERING?**	Bovine cough often present: • Refer urgently to Ear, Nose and Throat specialist for assessment of vocal cord function and consideration for Teflon injection of a vocal cord- tracheotomy is sometimes urgently required.
IS TREATMENT **APPROPRIATE?**	**Arrange definitive treatment:** • Contact clinical oncologist to consider urgent investigation and radiotherapy. Continue high dose dexamethasone until after radiotherapy. • Consider contacting chest specialist to consider urgent endoscopic insertion of bronchial stent.

NOTES

Superior vena caval vein obstruction is caused by tumour in the mediastinum preventing venous drainage from the head, arms and upper trunk. Usually this occurs over weeks or months, allowing alternative (collateral) drainage to develop, but occasionally the obstruction occurs rapidly over days and needs urgent treatment. Radiotherapy relieves symptoms in 50-95% within the first two weeks of treatment.[10] If radiotherapy is ineffective or cannot be used, a stent can be inserted into the SVC as a interventional radiology technique.

Stridor can be due to bilateral cord paralysis and needs referral to ENT specialists as severe obstruction can occur without warning, requiring a temporary tracheostomy. Otherwise the usual cause is external compression of the airway by tumour. A helium/oxygen mixture helps because its lower viscosity compared with air makes it easier to breathe.

Spinal cord compression in advanced cancer

Clinical decision	If YES → Action
Immediately **IS CORD COMPRESSION PRESENT OR A HIGH RISK?**	**Confirm presence or risk of compression:** • Early: vertebral pain (especially on coughing or lying); late: sensory changes, motor weakness; very late: sphincter disturbance. Sensory changes are usually one or two dermatomes below site of compression, except in cauda equina lesions where changes are often asymmetrical. **Start urgent treatment:** • If signs and symptoms are new (within 1 week) give dexamethasone 24mg IV as slow injection over 2 minutes. • Treat pain (see **Pain**) and manage urinary incontinence (see **Urinary problems**).
Within 24 hours **WILL PROGNOSIS ALLOW TIME FOR TREATMENT?**	**Establish diagnosis and arrange definitive treatment:** • Start dexamethasone 18mg PO daily in divided doses • *If deterioration is week by week or slower:* Contact clinical oncologist to consider urgent investigation and radiotherapy. • *If pain is persisting and severe:* ketamine or spinal analgesia (see **Emergencies**: severe pain)
Within 3 weeks **ARE NEUROLOGICAL SIGNS WORSENING?**	**Prevent deterioration in neurological function:** • Maintain dexamethasone at 18mg daily (as above). • If well enough, seek orthopaedic opinion for surgical decompression.
Within 6 weeks **HAS PERMANENT CORD DAMAGE OCCURRED?**	**Manage consequences of cord damage:** • See: **Constipation, Urinary problems**, and **Skin pressure** damage. Arrange for physiotherapy and occupational therapy. Contact rehabilitation medicine team for help and advice. • See: **the Anxious person, the Angry person, the Withdrawn patient**. • Reduce and stop dexamethasone (unless required for pain control).

NOTES

Cord compression requires prompt treatment- one third of patients survive at least a year after symptoms develop,[11] and patients deserve to be spared the distress of paraplegia if possible. Up to 5% of cancer patients may develop compression- this figure is higher in myeloma and prostatic carcinoma.[12] Back pain in a patient with cancer should alert the carer to the risk of compression- warning signs are radiating pain (unilateral in cervical or lumbar compression, bilateral in thoracic compression), unpleasant sensory changes in limbs, and pain on lying, coughing or straining. Sensory and motor loss occurs later, and sphincter disturbance is a late sign. The final stage is cord ischaemia that occurs rapidly over hours. High dose dexamethasone given immediately will reduce cord oedema and may temporarily prevent the onset of cord ischaemia. Radiotherapy is the definitive treatment. Surgery is worthwhile in suitable patients if radiotherapy is not possible, skeletal instability is present, or if the patient deteriorates whilst receiving dexamethasone and radiotherapy. Dexamethasone alone is suitable for patients for whom neither radiotherapy nor surgery is possible.

Diabetic emergencies in advanced disease

Clinical decision	If YES → Action

Immediately **IS URGENT TREATMENT REQUIRED?**	eg. drowsiness, confusion or coma
	Check blood glucose and start emergency treatment:
	• *If hypoglycaemic* (pale, sweaty, glucose<2.5mmol/l):
	  Give sugar in water orally, but if too sleepy give 20mls 50% glucose IV (flush needle with 0.9% saline to clear all glucose and prevent local thrombosis).
	  If IV access not available give glucagon 1mg IM.
	• *If hyperglycaemic* (glucose>15mmmol/l):
	  Start 28% oxygen (20% have a low O_2 saturation).
	  Check electrolytes, blood glucose and urinary ketones
	  Start up IV infusion 0.9% saline at 500ml/hour.

Within 1 hour **IS PATIENT STILL SYMPTOMATIC?**	**Stabilise condition:**
	• *If hypoglycaemic:* ensure glucose is being maintained above 5mmol/l. Repeat IV 20mls 50% glucose (or 1mg glucagon) if necessary.
	• *If hyperglycaemic:* - give 500mls 0.9% saline hourly until BP and peripheral circulation are normal and signs of dehydration have resolved.
	  Insulin: give short acting insulin 6 units IV **or** 20 units IM.
	  Potassium: 5 mins after first insulin give 13-20mmol/litre/hour with saline.
	  If hyperventilating: give 50 mmol bicarbonate + 10 mmol KCl in 30 mins.

Within 4 hours	**Maintain improvement:** • *If hypoglycaemic:* monitor glucose 4-hourly until 3 normal levels obtained. • *If hyperglycaemic:* give insulin 6 units/hour infusion IV or as hourly IM injections (SC cannot be used until peripheral circulation improves) Check blood glucose hourly, repeat electrolytes 1 and 5 hours after starting.

Within 24 hours	**Prevent recurrence** (see also **Diabetes in advanced disease**).
	• *Hypoglycaemia:* reduce dose of insulin or hypoglycaemics. Exclude other causes of hypoglycaemia (adrenocortical insufficiency, insulinomas, non-selective b-blockers, pentamidine, post gastrectomy dumping)
	• *Hyperglycaemia:* establish 24 hour requirement of insulin. Maintain glucose to whatever range controls symptoms (usually 8-15 mmol/l)
	  Convert to once daily insulin (eg. Ultratard).[15]
	  Exclude drug causes of hyperglycaemia (corticosteroids, octreotide, diuretics).

NOTES

Managing severe hypoglycaemia: symptoms will normally occur at glucose levels of less than 2mmol/l, although some patients with a history of hyperglycaemia may develop symptoms at higher levels up to 6mmol/l. Treatment should be immediate with glucose replacement. If there is any risk the patient may fail to swallow oral glucose because of drowsiness, 50% glucose should be given intravenously. If intravenous access is not possible, then 1mg glucagon can be given intramuscularly.

Managing severe hyperglycaemia:[13] Drowsiness, confusion or coma require urgent treatment. The main goals are to rehydrate, restore a normal BP, treat hypoxia, and reduce glucose while maintaining potassium levels. Both ketotic and non-ketotic hyperglycaemia can be treated in this way. Ketotic patients will be acidotic, and it is appropriate to treat this with sodium bicarbonate if they are hyperventilating, but in patients with advanced disease closer control is best done where blood gases and pH can be easily monitored. Glucose ranges of 8-15 mmol are acceptable as long as patients are asymptomatic. It is more important to avoid hypoglycaemia and the aim is to minimise symptoms, not the tight control of blood glucose.[14] Patients who have a history of hyperglycaemia may tolerate higher levels, and can develop hypoglycaemic symptoms at levels of 2-6mmol/l.

Emergencies:
NOTES AND REVISIONS (regular revision updates available on CLIP update service)

Emergencies:
NOTES AND REVISIONS (regular revision updates available on CLIP update service)

Drugs in palliative care for children

NB. Dosages for children are also given throughout the drug formulary.

Drug pharmacokinetics

Children absorb, distribute, metabolise and eliminate drugs differently to adults:

Neonates have a low renal and hepatic clearance with a higher volume of distribution. This prolongs the half-life of many drugs so that they require smaller doses relative to their size, but they may need a loading dose to avoid a delay in effect.

Infants and children: have relatively high clearances with a normal volume of distribution. This leads to shorter half lives compared with adults so that they may need comparatively higher doses at shorter intervals.

Drug presentation

Care and imagination are needed when selecting appropriate routes and preparations. Contrary to popular belief, children often prefer tablets to sickly sweet syrups. If liquids are used their taste can be improved with fizzy drinks or fruit juice. The rectal route provides effective and rapid absorption and some children are willing to self administer drugs this way. Subcutaneous infusions using portable, battery driven pumps (see <u>Syringe drivers</u>) are a valuable method of administering many drugs with minimum trouble to the child. Some children already have Hickman's venous access catheters in place often with several months experience of their use, providing an alternative route.

Drug	Oral starting dose		Parenteral or transdermal		Comments
	<50kg	>50kg	<50kg	>50kg	
Non-opioid primary analgesics: starting doses					
paracetamol	10mg/kg 6-hourly	10mg/kg 4-hourly	-	-	BNF recommends a max. of 4 doses in 24hours. Halve doses if jaundiced[1]
ibuprofen	5mg/kg 8-hourly	5-10mg/kg 8-hourly	-	-	Not for use in children under 7kg weight
diclofenac	500µg/kg 12-hourly	1mg/kg 12-hourly	-	-	Not for use in children under 12 months of age. Controlled release preparations not recommended for children.
Weak oral opioid primary analgesics: starting doses					
codeine	1mg/kg 4-6 hourly	60mg 3-4 hourly	-	-	Available as syrup.
dihydrocodeine	0.5mg/kg 4-6 hourly	30mg 3-4 hourly	-	-	Not recommended below 4 years

Drug	Oral starting dose		Parenteral or transdermal		Comments
	<50kg	>50kg	<50kg	>50kg	

Strong opioid primary analgesics (suggested starting doses for children not previously on strong opioids)

Drug	<50kg	>50kg	<50kg	>50kg	Comments
diamorphine	–	–	15 µg/kg/hr infusion	400 µg/hr infusion	Oral tablets available but no advantages over morphine
fentanyl (injection)	–	–	5 µg/hr infusion	10 µg/hr infusion	
fentanyl (transdermal)	–	–	Not suitable	25 µg/hr patch	25 µg/hr patch is smallest available. Complex pharma-cokinetics – see drug formulary
hydromorphone	20 µg/kg 4-6 hourly	3mg 3-4 hourly	3 µg/kg/hr infusion	150 µg/hr infusion	Not available in parenteral form in UK (as of Nov '97)
methadone	200 µg/kg 12-24 hrly	10mg 8-12 hourly	100 µg/kg 12-24 hourly	5mg 8-12 hourly	Special titration method required- see drug formulary
morphine (instant release)	160 µg/kg 4-6 hourly	7.5mg 3-4 hourly	20 µg/kg/hr infusion	1 mg/hr infusion	Can be made up in suppository form
morphine (controlled release)	500 µg/kg 12-hourly	25mg 8-12 hourly	–	–	Also available as suspension (MST Continus suspension)

Drug	Oral starting dose	Rectal, parenteral or transdermal	Comments

Secondary analgesics: starting doses

Drug	Oral starting dose	Rectal, parenteral or transdermal	Comments
amitriptyline	200 µg/kg once at night, titrated up to 1-2mg/kg if tolerated Syrup available.	Not recommended	Use with caution in children with cardiac dysfunction. Not recommended for depression.[1]
imipramine	0-7 years: not recommended >7: 1mg/kg.	–	Alternative to amitriptyline for neuropathic pain.
carbamazepine	1mg/kg 12-hourly	–	Syrup and 125mg suppositories available
hyoscine butylbromide	–	25 µg/kg/hr infusion	–
sodium valproate	5mg/kg 12-hourly	–	Syrup available

Drug	Oral starting dose	Rectal or parental or transdermal	Comments
Other drugs: starting doses			
baclofen	500 µg/kg daily Max doses: 1-2 years = 20mg; 3-6 years = 30mg; 7-10 years = 60mg	Not recommended	–
bisacodyl	5mg	–	–
carbamazepine	For seizures: Starting dose=1mg/kg 12-hourly; Maintenance for seizures up to 1 year =100-200mg; 1-5 years = 200-400mg; 5-10 years = 400-600mg, 10-15 years = 0.6 - 1g.	–	Syrup and 125mg suppositories available
carbocistiene	2-5 years = 62.5-125mg 6-hourly; 6-12 years = 250mg 8-hourly.	–	–
cisapride	0-11 = not recommended; >12 years 10-20mg 12-hourly	–	–
co-danthramer co-danthrusate	2.5 ml co-danthramer syrup or equivalent	–	Acceptable to use in life-threatening illness[3]
cyclizine	1-2 year = 1mg/kg 8-hourly; 2-12 years = 12.5mg 8-hourly	SC (as oral dose)	May cause local irritation given SC
desmopressin	PO = 100-200 microg.	SC = 0.5 - 1 microg. intranasal = 10-40 microg.	Can be used < 5 years for diabetes insipidus.
dexamethasone	Starting doses same as adult	SC (as for oral dose)	Reduce to lowest dose that controls symptoms
diazepam	200 microg./kg 4-6 hourly.	For seizure PR: 500 microg./kg repeated if necessary or slow IV injection: 250 microg./kg.	Maximum 10mg as a single dose. Rectal route preferred.
dimethicone (dimeticone)	20-40mg with each feed.	–	See drug formulary for available preparations
docusate	–	5ml rectal solution as required	Oral solution no longer available.
domperidone	200-400 microg./kg 4-8 hourly.	PR 10-15kg = 15mg 12-hrly; 15.5-25kg = 30mg 12-hrly; 25.5-35kg = 30mg 8-hrly; 35.5-45kg = 30mg 6-hrly.	
fluconazole	3-6mg/kg (daily if >1 month, once every 48-72 hrs if < 1month)	IV (as for oral dose)	–
frusemide	1-3mg/kg daily	IM or slow IV: 0.5-1.5 mg/kg. Max 20mg daily	–

85

Drug	Oral starting dose	Rectal, parenteral or transdermal	Comments
Other drugs: starting doses			
glycopyrronium	–	5µg/kg/ or 0.5 µg/kg/hr infusion	Alternative to hyoscine hydrobromide
haloperidol	10-25 microg./kg 12-hourly. Only lowest doses required for nausea.	SC (as for oral dose)	Avoid high doses or prolonged courses if possible.
hyoscine butylbromide	–	25µg/kg/hr SC infusion	Less sedating alternative to glycopyrronium
hyoscine hydrobromide (tablets, injection)	5µg/kg 6-hourly	5 µg/kg. as SC single dose (or 1µg/kg/hr infusion).	More sedating than glycopyrronium.
hyoscine hydrobromide (transdermal)	–	<4 years = half patch (~75µg/24 hours) >4 years =whole patch	Found to be useful in paediatric palliative care[3]
ketoconazole	3mg/kg once daily	–	–
levomepromazine (methotrimeprazine)	Antiemetic:100µg./kg 12 hourly Sedation: 250 µg/kg 4-8 hourly	As oral doses or 0.5-3mg/ kg/24 hours SC infusion for sedation	Found to be useful in paediatric palliative care[3]
loperamide	0-4 years = not recommended; 4-12 years = 1mg up to 6-hourly.	–	In acute infection, 3-5 days use only.
metoclopramide	up to 10kg = 1mg 12-hourly; 10-14kg = 1mg 8-12 hourly; 15-19kg = 2mg 8-12 hourly; 20-29kg = 2.5mg 8-hourly; >30kg = 5mg 8-hourly.	As for oral dose	Daily doses should not exceed 500 µg/kg
metronidazole	7.5mg/kg 8-hourly	IV as for oral route	–
midazolam	–	20-100 µg/kg/hr infusion	Gives much finer control than diazepam
paraldehyde		0.3ml/kg PR (max10 mls)	Mix with arachis oil 1:1
phenobarbital	=	15mg/kg SC/IV single dose or 500µg/kg/hr SC infusion	–
ranitidine	2-4mg/kg 12-hourly	–	Daily doses should not exceed 300mg.
spironolactone	1-1.5mg/kg	–	
sucralfate	1-2 g swallowed or topical	–	Used as a haemostatic agent or gastric mucosal coating agent
tranexamic acid	30mg/kg 8-hourly	–	Can be used topically to stop bleeding

Children: NOTES AND REVISIONS (regular revision updates available on CLIP update service)

Prescribing in the last hours and days

As patients become semiconscious and unable to take drugs by mouth, radical revision of medication requirements is mandatory. The rectal and subcutaneous routes can be utilised in the majority of instances. Although many patients will no longer be given drugs by mouth, oral hygiene will continue to be an important part of overall care.

Rationalising drugs in the last hours and days		
Drug	**Suggested action**	**Alternative action**
Analgesics		
paracetamol	stop	paracetamol 500mg PR
weak opioids	diamorphine SC 2.5-5mg PRN	diamorphine SC infusion
strong opioids	diamorphine at equivalent doses	transdermal fentanyl (will need at least 12 hours diamorphine cover on starting)
NSAIDs eg naproxen	stop	diclofenac 100mg PR once daily
Corticosteroids		
eg. dexamethasone injection/infusion	stop	if used as co-analgesic give as SC infusion
Laxatives		
eg. co-danthramer	stop	-
Antiemetics		
haloperidol	continue by SC injection once at night	levomepromazine SC
cyclizine	continue by SC injection or infusion	cyclizine PR
metoclopramide	continue by SC injection or infusion	domperidone PR
hyoscine hydrobromide	continue by SC injection or infusion	transdermal hyoscine hydrobromide
levomepromazine	continue by SC injection or infusion	chlorpromazine PR
Psychotropic drugs		
antidepressants	stop	-
benzodiazepines	midazolam as SC infusion	diazepam PR
haloperidol	continue by SC injection or infusion	levomepromazine SC
levomepromazine (methotrimeprazine)	continue by SC injection or infusion	chlorpromazine PR
Anticonvulsants		
eg. phenytoin, valproate	carbamazepine PR once daily	phenobarbital SC once daily
Antimicrobial agents		
eg. amoxycillin	stop	hyoscine hydrobromide for excess bronchial secretions
Cardiovascular and endocrine drugs		
eg. frusemide, insulin	stop	-
Miscellaneous		
baclofen	replace with diazepam PR	midazolam SC infusion
dantrolene	stop	midazolam SC infusion
bronchodilators	stop	hyoscine/atropine SC PRN
enteral nutrition	stop	-
wound management	minimise dressing changes	-

Drug formulary

NP = non-proprietary drug supplied from one or more manufacturers without a trade name.
IM = intramuscular; IV = intravenous; PO = oral; PR = rectal; SC = subcutaneous; SL = sublingual.
Numbers refer to British National Formulary and Palliative Care Formulary. [1, 85]

amitriptyline
(4.3.1. Tricyclic and related antidepressant drugs)
PO, IM.

Preparations: tablets (NP, Domical, Elavil, Tryptizol); capsules (Lentizol); solution (NP, Triptyzol); injection (Tryptizol).

Indications: neuropathic pain (low dose), depression (standard dose).

Action: strong inhibition of presynaptic uptake of serotonin and some inhibition of noradrenaline uptake.

Dose: start with 25mg at night (10mg in elderly) and titrate weekly up to 50-150mg.

Children: [1, 2] For depression: not recommended. For neuropathic pain: 200 microg./kg PO once at night, titrated up to 1-2mg/kg if needed. For enuresis: 7-10 years = 10-20mg PO at night; 11-16 years = 25-50mg PO at night. Injection: not recommended.

Contraindications: recent myocardial infarction, heart block, porphyria, mania, severe liver impairment. Use with caution in patients with narrow angle glaucoma, urinary retention or hypotension.

Common adverse effects: usual antimuscarinic effects: dry mouth, blurred vision, urinary retention, constipation, difficulty in visual accommodation, ileus, increased ocular pressure, sedation, tachycardia, postural hypotension, sweating.

Interactions: adverse effects of amitriptyline increased with nefopam, phenothiazines and cimetidine; do not give within 2 weeks treatment with MAOIs (monoamine oxidase inhibitors); *reduces the actions of* anti-epileptics; *increases the actions* of baclofen.

Comments: some elderly patients will not tolerate starting doses above 10mg at night. Increase gradually as tolerated. Give as single night time dose to minimise impact of sedative and antimuscarinic effects. Effective in neuropathic pain [46, 48] regardless of the pattern of pain. [47]

baclofen
(10.2.2. Skeletal muscle relaxants)
PO, spinal.

Preparations: tablets (NP, Baclospas, Baglifen, Lioresal); solution (Lioresal); intrathecal injection (Lioresal).

Indications: skeletal muscle spasm; hiccup.

Action: stimulation of presynaptic $GABA_B$ receptors, which are inhibitory receptors.

Dose: start at 5mg 8-hourly after food to minimise nausea and drowsiness. Usual max.100mg daily.

Children: [1, 3] starting dose PO- 500 microg./kg daily; maintenance 1-2 years = 10-20mg daily; 3-6 years = 20-30mg daily; 7-10 years = 30-60mg daily. Injection: not recommended.

Contraindications: peptic ulceration, will potentiate effects of antihypertensive treatment; may exacerbate psychotic states and epilepsy.

Common adverse effects: nausea, daytime sedation. Abrupt withdrawal can cause autonomic dysreflexia-dose should be reduced over at least 1-2 weeks.

Interactions: adverse effects of baclofen increased by tricyclic antidepressants, NSAIDs, β-blockers, nifedipine, and lithium; *effects of baclofen reduced by* carbamazepine and phenytoin.

Comments: liquid available. Intrathecal route occasionally used after intractable spasticity when oral route produces intolerable adverse effects.

bisacodyl

PO, PR.

Preparations: tablets (NP, Dulco-lax); suppositories (NP).

Indications: constipation.

Action: contact stimulant acting on small and large bowel.

Dose:[1] 5-10mg at night or twice daily PO; 10-20mg once daily PR.

Children: 5mg at night.

Contraindications: intestinal obstruction.

Common adverse effects: suppositories may produce a burning sensation in the rectum. Mild proctitis can occur on prolonged use.

Comments: tablets act in 10 to 12 hours; suppositories in 20 to 60 minutes. Do not chew. Do take within one hour of antacids or milk.

Brompton Cocktail

Not recommended for use

Mixtures containing morphine or diamorphine in fixed combinations with cocaine, phenothiazines and alcohol have no advantages over simple morphine solutions.[4-6]

---

bupivacaine

SC, IM, spinal

Preparations: injection (Marcaine).

Indications: longer acting nerve block (procedures, spinal, peripheral nerve block).

Action: inhibition of neural transmission.

Dose: intrathecal = see section on spinal analgesia; peripheral block = up to 30 mL 0.5% or 60ml 0.25%.

Children: no information.

Contraindications: do not use in patients who are sensitive to amide anaesthetic agents.

Common adverse effects: after high doses or after inadvertent intravascular injection, hypotension, myocardial, depression and a variety of CNS effects can occur.

Interactions: use of beta blockers and local anaesthetics containing adrenaline may enhance sympathomimetic side effects.

---

buprenorphine

SL, IM, IV

Preparations: tablets (Temgesic); injection (Temgesic).

Indications: opioid-sensitive pain.

Action: partial stimulation of opioid *mu* receptors and *delta* opioid receptors, blocking of *kappa* opioid receptors.

Dose: 200-400 microg. 8-hourly.

Children:[1] 0-6 months: not recommended; above 6 months = 3-6 microg./kg (max. 9microg/kg).

Contraindications: no absolute contraindications in patients with advanced and progressing disease.

Common adverse effects: on initiating treatment some patients are troubled with drowsiness, nausea or confusion, hypotension and sweating. With continuing treatment, constipation occurs in many patients and small pupils are common.

Interactions: *adverse effects enhanced by* other CNS depressants and cimetidine; *reduces the action of* mexiletine; hypertension or hypotension may occur with MAOIs.

Comments: no clear advantages over morphine/diamorphine or alternatives such as hydromorphone.

carbamazepine
PO, PR.

Preparations: tablets (NP, Epimaz, Tegretol, Tegretol Retard); solution (Tegretol); suppositories (Tegretol).
Indications: neuropathic pain, seizures (except absence seizures).
Action: possibly through stabilising cell membranes and by enhancing GABA inhibition of synaptic transmission.
Dose: 100 to 800mg daily, occasionally up to 600mg 12-hourly.
Children: starting dose = 2mg/kg PO 6 hourly. Maintenance for seizures up to 1 year =100-200mg; 1-5 years = 200-400mg; 5-10 years = 400-600mg, 10-15 years = 0.6 - 1g.
Contraindications: do not use in patients with A-V conduction abnormalities unless paced.
Common adverse effects: nausea, vomiting, dizziness, drowsiness, headache, ataxia, confusion, agitation, visual disturbances, constipation, diarrhoea, anorexia, transient erythematous rash, leucopaenia.
Interactions: effect enhanced by dextropropoxyphene, erythromycin, fluoxetine, diltiazem, cimetidine; *effect reduced* by antidepressants and danazol; *carbamazepine reduces the effect of* warfarin, digoxin, tricyclics, haloperidol, corticosteroids, tramadol, thyroid hormones and doxycycline. Variable effects of carbamazepine are seen with theophylline and phenytoin.
Comments: autoinduction reduces half-life from about 36 hours initially to 16-24 hours on chronic dosing. Start with low, frequent dose eg. 50mg 6-hourly.

---

carbocisteine
PO

Preparations: capsules (NP, Mucodyne); liquid (NP, Mucodyne).
Indications: thick sputum.
Action: reduces sputum viscosity.
Dose: 500-750mg 8-hourly.
Children: 2-5 years = 62.5-125mg 6-hourly; 6-12 years = 250mg 8-hourly.
Contraindications: active peptic ulceration.
Common adverse effects: GI irritation, rashes.
Interactions: none.
Comments: has been used in patients with cystic fibrosis.

---

cisapride
PO

Preparations: tablets (Prepulsid); suspension (Prepulsid).
Indications: reduced gastric motility not responding to domperidone or metoclopramide; reduced bowel motility.
Action: $5HT_4$ agonist speeding gastric, small bowel and large bowel transit.[7]
Dose: 10mg 8-hourly or 20mg 12-hourly.
Children: not recommended below 12 years. Above 12 years as adult doses.
Contraindications: do not use with grapefruit juice.
Common adverse effects: abdominal cramp, diarrhoea.
Interactions: effects enhanced by erythromycin, ketoconazole, ibraconazole, miconazole and fluconazole (with risk of ventricular arryhthmias); *cisapride increases the effects of* oral anticoagulants.
Comments: More potent than domperidone or metoclopramide.

clonidine   *(2.5.1. Vasodilator antihypertensive drugs)*

PO, spinal.

Preparations: tablets (Catapres); capsules (Catapres Perlongets); injection (Catapres).

Indications: neuropathic pain.

Action: as spinal analgesic: α_2 - adrenergic agonist causing spinal cholinergic activation; enhancement of local anaesthetic action.[8]

Dose: 150 micrograms 8-hourly by mouth; 50 - 150 micrograms per 24 hours intrathecally.

Children: no information available.

Contraindications: no absolute contraindications.

Common adverse effects: dry mouth, sedation, depression, fluid retention, bradycardia, Raynaud's phenomenon, headache, dizziness, euphoria, nocturnal unrest, rash, nausea, constipation.

Interactions: Clonidine may inhibit antiparkinsonian effect of levodopa.

Comments: following sudden withdrawal, rebound hypertension may be exacerbated by concurrent beta blocker or tricyclic antidepressant therapy.

---

co-danthramer/co-danthramer forte suspensions   *(1.6.2. Stimulant laxatives)*

PO.

Preparations: capsules (NP); suspension (Ailax, Ailax Forte, Codalax, Codalax Forte).

Indications: constipation.

Action: contact colonic stimulant (danthron) with wetting agent (poloxamer).

Dose: titrated to individual patient to produce comfortable stool without colic.

Children: can be used in children with life-threatening illness in same doses as adults.[3] Preferable to lactulose which causes bloating and abdominal discomfort

Contraindications: bowel obstruction.

Common adverse effects: Colic, urine may be coloured red, some patients have irritation and excoriation around perineum producing reddish brown rash around perineum (due to danthron staining and sensitivity).

Comments: contains poloxamer as softener + danthron as contact stimulant. 5ml co-danthramer syrup contains 25mg danthron + 200mg poloxamer '188'; 5ml co-danthramer forte contains 75mg danthron + 1 gram poloxamer '188'.

---

co-danthrusate   *(1.6.2. Stimulant laxatives)*

PO.

Preparations: capsules (Capsuvac, Normax); suspension (Normax).

Indications: constipation.

Action: contact colonic stimulant (danthron) with wetting agent (docusate).

Dose: titrated to individual patient to produce a comfortable stool without colic. Usual range 1-9 capsules per day).

Children: can be used in children with life-threatening illness in same doses as adults.[3] Preferable to lactulose which causes bloating and abdominal discomfort

Contraindications: intestinal obstruction.

Common adverse effects: as for co-danthramer.

Comments: each capsule contains 50mg danthron and 60mg docusate sodium.

codeine

PO, IM, SC, IV.

Preparations: tablets (NP); solution (NP); injection (NP).
Indications: mild, opioid-sensitive pain.
Action: weak stimulation of opioid *mu* receptors.
Dose: 15 to 60mg 4-hourly.
Children: [1,2] PO starting doses: <50kg = 1mg/kg 4-6 hourly; >50kg = 60mg 3-4 hourly.
Contraindications: no absolute contraindications in patients with advanced disease.
Common adverse effects: on initiating treatment some patients are troubled with drowsiness, nausea or confusion. With continuing treatment, constipation occurs in many patients and small pupils are common.
Interactions: as for morphine.
Comments: Has the same dose-response relationship as morphine so that the same analgesic effect requires more drug (mg for mg) but, like other weak opioids, it is more likely to produce adverse effects. This limits its use in advanced disease such that, if strong opioids are easily available, there is no advantage in using weak opioids alone.[9] Usually supplied as the phosphate salt. About one-tenth as potent as morphine. Excreted mainly by the kidney as conjugates of glucuronic acid. Half-life is 3 to 4 hours.

cyclizine

PO, PR, IM, SC.

Preparations: tablets (Valoid); injection (Valoid). Suppositories can be made by special order.
Indications: vagally-mediated nausea or vomiting.
Action (presumed): histamine and cholinergic receptor antagonist at vomiting centres.
Dose: 25- 50mg every 8 hours or 75-150mg / 24 hours SC infusion.
Children: 1-2 years = 1mg/kg 8-hourly; 2-12 years = 12.5 - 25mg 8-hourly.
Contraindications: no absolute contraindications in patients with advanced disease.
Common adverse effects: drowsiness, dry mouth, blurred vision, hypotension.
Interactions: adverse effects increased by tricyclic antidepressants, haloperidol and metoclopramide. Solutions of diamorphine and cyclizine are incompatible at concentrations of either drug >25mg/ml (higher diamorphine concentrations can be used if cyclizine concentration is kept to 10mg/ml or less). These drugs are also incompatible in solutions where pH > 8.

dantrolene

(10.2.2) PO, IV.

Preparations: capsules (Dantrium); injection (Dantrium).
Indications: skeletal muscle spasm.
Action: acts directly on skeletal muscle to produce relaxation.
Dose: Start with 25mg daily. Titrate up to 25-75mg 6-hourly.
Children: [1] not recommended.
Contraindications: severe hepatic dysfunction, acute muscle spasm.
Common adverse effects: drowsiness, dizziness, weakness, malaise, fatigue, diarrhoea, anorexia, nausea, headache, rash.
Interactions: adverse effects of dantrolene increased by tricyclic antidepressants, NSAIDs, β-blockers, nifedipine, and lithium; *effects of dantrolene reduced by* carbamazepine and phenytoin.
Interactions: Use with verapamil may cause hyperkalaemia.
Comments: monitor hepatic function. Increase dose slowly at weekly intervals.

desmopressin
(6.5.2. Posterior pituitary hormones and antagonists)

PO, SC, intranasally, IM, IV.

Preparations: tablets (DDVAP, Desmotabs); nasal spray (DDVAP, Desmospray); injection (DDVAP).

Indications: diabetes insipidus, intractable nocturnal incontinence of urine.

Action: increased permeability of distal convoluted tubules and collecting ducts of the kidneys, resulting in increased water resorption and reduced urine volume.

Dose:[1] PO = 100-200 microg.; intranasal = 10-40 microg. SC = 0.5 - 1 microg. Give 8-hourly for diabetes insipidus and once at night for incontinence.

Children: same as adult doses. Not recommended below 5 years for incontinence.

Contraindications: cardiovascular disease; renal impairment, hypertension, cystic fibrosis.

Common adverse effects: fluid retention, hyponatraemia.

Interactions: Increased effect of desmopressin by indomethacin, carbamazepine, hithium, chlorpropamide.

Comments: use with care in cases where water retention could be a problem. Avoid in cystic fibrosis.

dexamethasone
(6.3.2. Glucocorticoid therapy)

PO, SC, IM, IV.

Preparations: tablets (NP, Decadron); injection (Decadron). Tablets disperse easily in water.

Indications: high dose (8-24mg daily)- peritumour oedema; low dose (2-6mg daily)- anorexia, lethargy.

Action: In oedema may reduce capillary permeability- other action poorly understood.

Dose: 2mg to 16mg daily in single or divided doses.

Children:[2] starting doses same as adult, maintaining on lowest dose to control symptoms.

Contraindications: systemic fungal infection.

Common adverse effects: hypokalaemia, adrenal suppression, weight gain, Cushing's syndrome, hyperglycaemia, well being, insomnia, osteoporosis, impaired wound healing, myopathy.

Interactions: Effects increased by diuretics (hypokalaemia), NSAIDs (GI bleeding); *effects reduced by* aminoglutethamide, barbiturates, carbamazepine, cholestyramine, cyclophosphamide, phenytoin, phenobarbitone, primidone and rifampicin. Steroids may affect prothrombinaemic response to warfarin. Enhances excretion of salicylate.

Comments: parenteral dose is half to one third of oral dose. Benefit can sometimes be obtained on going higher than 16mg in cerebral tumours.[10, 11] The belief that steroids increase peptic ulceration or GI bleeding is based on weak evidence. [49, 50] We do not routinely cover patients on corticosteroids unless they are concurrently on NSAID's, have taken a cummulative dose of 40mg or more, or have a previous history of ulceration.

dextromoramide
(4.7.2. Opioid analgesics)

PO, PR

Preparations: tablets (Palfium); suppositories (Palfium).

Indications: opioid-sensitive pain; possible use as breakthrough medication during transdermal fentanyl administration.

Action: stimulation of opioid *mu-* receptors.

Dose: titrated to individual needs (starting dose 5mg).

Children: no information.

Contraindications: no absolute contraindications in patients with advanced disease.

Common adverse effects: as for morphine.

Comments: is approximately twice as potent as morphine and is given orally or rectally. The sublingual route may be less predictable.[12] Has a similar structure to fentanyl and, in our experience, is useful for breakthrough pain in patients taking fentanyl.

diamorphine

(PO, SC, IM, IV)

Preparations: tablets (NP); injection (NP).
Indications: opioid-sensitive pain.
Action: no intrinsic activity (converted to morphine)
Dose: 5mg to 5000mg daily SC 4-hourly, or as SC infusion.
Children:[2] <50kg = 15 microg./kg/hr infusion; >50kg = 400 microg./hr infusion.
Contraindications: no absolute contraindications in patients with advanced and progressing disease.
Common adverse effects: as for morphine.
Interaction: as for morphine.
Comments: depressant effects are enhanced by other CNS depressants. GI effects may alter the rate of absorption of other drugs. Use with caution in patients with impaired renal function or hypothyroidism. Diamorphine is as effective as morphine,[13] and there is no evidence that regular oral medication with one has any advantages over the other. This is not surprising since diamorphine is a prodrug for morphine.[14] Oral morphine and diamorphine appear to be equipotent, but parenteral diamorphine is twice as potent as parenteral morphine.[85]

diazepam

PO, PR, IV.

Preparations: tablets (NP, Atenesine, Rimapam, Tensium, Valium); solution (Dialar, Valium); rectal (Rectubes, Stesolid, Valclair); injection (Diazemuls, Valium).
Indications: acute control of major seizure or catastrophic situation (eg. major bleed). Sedation where long acting drug is needed.
Action: facilitation of GABA binding to GABA receptors.
Dose: 2 to 20mg as a single dose. Titrate IV doses slowly (initially 1-2mg/min if requirements are unknown) unless sedation is needed for an emergency in which case titration can be faster. Catastrophic bleeding is the only situation in which it is acceptable to give a 10-20mg bolus IV.
Children:[1,2] PO: 200 microg./kg 4-6 hourly. For seizure PR: 500 microg./kg repeated as necessary or slow IV injection: 250 microg./kg. Maximum 10mg as a single dose. Rectal route is preferred to IV.
Contraindications: acute pulmonary insufficiency.
Common adverse effects: drowsiness, light-headedness, confusion, ataxia, amnesia, paradoxical agitation. Respiratory depression is a risk if given IV. Local phlebitis (reduced with emulsion).
Interactions: *increased adverse effect* with isoniazid, CNS depressants, baclofen, nabilone, cimetidine, omeprazole.
Comments: Use with caution in elderly patients since their half life may be 7 days or more, creating uncertainty whether a patient is ill because of the advanced disease itself or the diazepam.

diclofenac
(10.1.1. Non-steroidal anti-inflammatory drugs)

PO, PR, IM, topical.

Preparations: tablets (NP, Dexomon, Dicloflex, Diclotard, Diclozip, Enzed, Flamrase, Lofensaid, Rheumalgan, Slofenac, Volsaid Retard, Valenac, Volraman, Voltarol, Voltarol Retard, Voltarol SR); capsules (Diclomax SR, Diclomax Retard, Motifene); suppositories (Voltarol); injection (NP, Voltarol); topical (Voltarol Emugel).

Indications: pain due to inflammation; bone pain unresponsive to opioids whilst awaiting other treatments.

Action: inhibition of cyclo-oxygenase (COX).

Dose: up to 50mg 8-hourly. Slow release tabs. containing 75mg and 100mg available.

Children:[1] <1 year = not recommended; 1-12 years = 0.5-1mg/kg 12-hourly. Controlled release preparations are not recommended for children.

Contraindications: active peptic ulcer or GI bleeding; thrombocytopaenia; asthmatic patients in whom NSAIDs cause asthma, urticaria or acute rhinitis. Do not use suppositories in patients with acute inflammatory condition of anus, rectum or sigmoid colon. Use with caution in patients taking anticoagulants.

Common adverse effects: at initiation of therapy: epigastric pain, nausea, diarrhoea, headache, slight dizziness. GI ulceration with melaena and/or haematemesis are a major risk, especially in ill patients. *NB: H_2 antagonists do not prevent gastric ulceration due to NSAIDs as ibuprofen.* Itching, burning and increased frequency of bowel movement after suppositories. Injections may cause abscesses if given into thigh.

Interactions: diclofenac adverse effects increased by diuretics (nephrotoxicity); *increases the adverse effects* of warfarin, sulphonylureas, phenytoin, corticosteroids (GI bleeding and ulceration), lithium, baclofen. Avoid NSAIDs in patients receiving antineoplastic doses of methotrexate. If gastric protection is necessary, use misoprostol.

Comments: NSAIDs usually inhibit renal clearance of lithium. Decrease dose in severe renal failure.

---

dihydrocodeine
(4.7.2. Opioid analgesics)

PO, IM.

Preparations: tablets (NP, DF118, DF118, DHC Continus).

Indications: mild opioid-sensitive pain.

Action: weak stimulation of opioid *mu*-receptors.

Dose: 30-60 mg 4-hourly by mouth or 60-120mg 12 hourly using S/R tablet.

Children:[1] PO starting doses: 0-4 years = not recommended; <50kg = 500 microg./kg 4-6 hourly; >50kg = 30mg 3-4 hourly.

Contraindications: no absolute contraindications in patients with advanced disease.

Common adverse effects : as for morphine.

Interactions: as for morphine.

Comments: about one tenth as potent as morphine. Has the same dose-response relationship as morphine the same analgesic effect requires more drug (mg for mg) so, like other weak opioids, it is more likely to produce adverse effects. This limits its use in disease such that, if strong opioids are easily available, there is no advantage in using weak opioids alone.[9]

dimeticone (dimethicone)
(1.1. Antacids and other drugs for dyspepsia)
PO

Preparations: Dentinox emulsion (42mg/5ml), Infacol liquid (200mg/5ml), Windcheater capsules. The following contain dimethicone: Asilone suspension (135mg/5ml), Diovol suspension (25mg/5ml), Maalox Plus suspension (25mg/5ml), Actonorm Gel, Altacite Plus tablets, Aslione tablets, Bisadol Extra tablets, Simeco, Sovol, Unigest.
Action: surface active agent which disperses foam and allows gastric air to be brought up.
Dose: 100-200mg 4-hourly.
Children:[1] 20-40mg with each feed.
Contraindications: no absolute contraindications in patients with advanced disease.
Common adverse effects : none.

---

dipipanone with cyclizine
Not recommended for use in advanced disease.
Sedation caused by the 30mg cyclizine in each tablet limits dose increases.

---

docusate/dioctyl
(1.6.2. Stimulant laxatives)
PO.

Preparations: capsules (Dioctyl); rectal solution (Fletcher's Enemette, Nogalax Micro-enema). See also co-danthrusate.
Indications: mild constipation; prevention of constipation in presence of partial bowel obstruction.
Action: wetting agent and mild contact stimulant acting on small and large bowel.
Dose: up to 200 mg 8-hourly.
Children: an oral solution is no longer available. Only the rectal solutions are suitable for use in children.
Contraindications: total intestinal obstruction; concurrent use of liquid paraffin.
Common adverse effects: colic, burning in throat after doses of liquid preparation.
Comments: acts as faecal softener by allowing water to penetrate desiccated faeces.

---

domperidone
(4.6. Drugs used in nausea and vertigo)
PO, PR.

Preparations: tablets (Motilium); suspension (Motilium); suppositories (Motilium).
Indications: reduced gastric motility.
Action: dopamine antagonist speeding gastric emtying.[7]
Dose: 10 to 20mg PO 12-hourly; 30 to 60mg PR 8-hourly.
Children: PO 200-400 microg./kg 4-8 hourly. PR 10-15kg = 15 12-hourly; 15.5-25kg = 30mg 12-hourly; 25.5-35kg = 30mg 8-hourly; 35.5-45kg = 30mg 6-hourly.
Contraindications: total intestinal obstruction.
Interactions: *effects of domperidone reduced by* opioid analgesics.
Common adverse effects: raised prolactin may cause galactorrhoea & gynaecomastia.
Comments: decreased incidence of extrapyramidal reactions as low propensity to cross the blood-brain barrier.

ethamsylate

PO, IM, IV, topical.

Preparations: tablets (Dicynene); injection (Dicynene).

Indications: capillary bleeding; haematuria.

Action (presumed): corrects abnormal platelet adhesion and decreases capillary fragility.

Dose: 500mg 6-hourly after food.

Children: no information.

Contraindications: porphyria.

Common adverse effects: nausea, headache, rashes.

Comments: rapidly absorbed orally and excreted unchanged in the bladder. Adverse effects are less troublesome than with tranexamic acid. Has been described as effective topically.

fentanyl (transdermal)
(4.7.2. Opioid analgesics)

Transdermal

Preparations: transdermal patches (Durgesic).

Indications: intolerable morphine adverse effects; pain in presence of renal failure.

Action: strong stimulation of opioid *mu*-receptors.

Dose: 25 - 500 microg/hour. Smaller dose rates (<25µg/hr) have to be given by SC infusion.

Children: has been used on children.

Contraindications: pyrexia or erythema (increases absorption); sweating (prevents adhesion);[15, 16] opioid-naive (ie. not previously on opioid).

Common adverse effects. Constipation and sedation are less troublesome than with morphine, but the pain relief and quality of life are the same.[17] Opioid hyperexcitability is a risk as it is with morphine.[18]

Interactions: adverse effects enhanced by other CNS depressants and cimetidine; *reduces the action of* mexiletine; hypertension or hypotension may occur with MAOIs.

Comments: depressant effects are enhanced by other CNS depressants. There is a slow onset of action (4-48 hours)[19, 20] and patients will need additional analgesia for up to 24 hours. There is also a slow elimination (up to 31 hours).[20, 21] Because of the delayed onset of fentanyl, the last dose of morphine (ideally as controlled release morphine), should be given when the patch is applied. This also reduces the likelihood of an opioid withdrawal syndrome which can occur on switching to fentanyl. [82] Laxatives should be stopped 24 hours before changing to fentanyl and then retitrated afterwards. Although the system appears to be safe and effective in cancer pain,[22] it is more complicated to use than oral morphine. Transdermal fentanyl is useful when adverse effects of other opioids prevent titration to an adequate dose or when renal problems are causing accumulation of M6G and M3G.

A quick conversion rule: oral morphine (mg / 24hrs) ÷ 3 = transdermal fentanyl (microg / hr)

parenteral diamorphine (mg / 24 hrs) = transdermal fentanyl (microg / hr)

This rule ensures that correct doses can be easily and quickly checked. Compared with the manufacturers dosing tables, this quick conversion results in a slightly higher dose of fentanyl on converting from morphine, and a slightly lower dose of morphine on converting from fentanyl (see overleaf). This may be appropriate as there are suggestions that fentanyl is less potent than suggested by the manufacturers.[23]

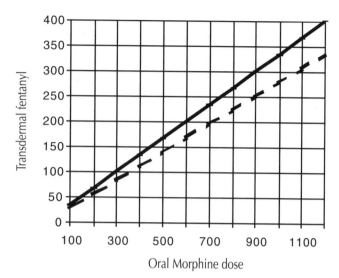

Fentanyl conversion
Comparison between manufacturer's conversion recommendations and quick conversion calculation.

Quick conversion ——

Manufacturer's ▬ ▬

(Graph axes: Transdermal fentanyl (y-axis, 0 to 400); Oral Morphine dose (x-axis, 100 to 1100))

---

fluconazole
(5.2. Antifungal drugs)
PO, IV.
Preparations: capsules (Diflucan); suspension (Diflucan); injection (Diflucan).
Indication: candidal infection in advanced disease.
Action: antifungal.
Dose: 150mg stat for candidosis in vagina or mouth; 14 to 30 days for oesophagitis or candiduria.
Children: neonate = 3-6mg/kg. once every 48-72 hours. Older children = 3-6mg/kg daily.
Contraindications: no absolute contraindications.
Common adverse effects: nausea, abdominal discomfort, flatulence.
Interactions: action of fluconazole reduced by antimuscarinics, rifampicin; *action of fluconazole increased by* hydrochlorthiazide; *fluconazole increase the action of* warfarin, sulphonylureas, phenytoin, midazolam; cisapride (risk of ventricular arryhthmias), tolbulamide, glipizide.

---

furosomide (frusemide)
(2.2.2. Loop diuretics)
PO, IV, IM.
Preparations: tablets (NP, Dryptal, Froop, Lasix); solution (Lasix); injection (NP, Lasix).
Indications: acute ventricular failure; malignant ascites (with spironolactone).
Action: inhibition of chloride transport in the ascending loop of Henle, increasing urinary sodium with resultant increase in urine volume.
Dose: 40 to 80mg daily, as a single dose in the morning or twice daily. If IV give slowly (4mg/min).
Children: [1] PO: 1-3mg/kg daily. IM or slow IV: 0.5-1.5mg/kg (max 20mg daily).
Contraindications: anuria; use with care in prostatic hypertrophy and impairment of micturition.
Common adverse effects: hyponatraemia, hypokalaemia, hypomagnesaemia, alkalosis, hypotension.
Interactions: increases the adverse effects of NSAIDs (renal damage, especially indomethacin), tricyclic antidepressants (hypotension), carbamazepine (hyponatraemia), corticosteroids (hypokalaemia); *reduces the action of* oral hypoglycaemics, risk of hypokalaemia increased by concurrent steroid therapy.

glycopyrrolate

(15.1.3. Antimuscarinic drugs)

SC, IM

Preparations: injection (Robinul).

Indications: troublesome bronchial secretions; inoperable bowel obstruction.

Action: antimuscarinic.

Dose: 200-400 microg. 2-hourly as required or 600 - 1200 microg. SC infusion per 24 hours.

Children:[1] 5 microg./kg. as single dose (or 0.5microg./kg/hr infusion).

Contraindications: in long-term use- closed angle glaucoma. No absolute contraindications for managing bronchial secretions in the last hours and days of life.

Common adverse effects: tachycardia, drowsiness, dry mouth, blurred vision, flushed face, amnesia; central stimulation may precede depression, urinary retention, may worsen existing cardiac insufficiency.

Interactions: as for hyoscine hydrobromide.

Comments: a fraction of the cost of hyoscine hydrobromide.

haloperidol

(4.2.1. Antipsychotic drugs)

PO, SC, IM, IV.

Preparations: tablets (NP, Haldol, Serenace); capsules (Serenace); solution (Dozic, Haldol, Serenace); injection (Haldol, Serenace).

Indications: chemical causes of emesis; acute confusional states.

Action: dopamine antagonist.

Dose: chemical causes of vomiting – 1.5-3mg nocte; control of acute confusional state – 5mg (1.5-3mg in elderly) PO/SC repeated as necessary (up to 30mg in 24 hours).

Children:[1,2] 10-25 microg./kg 12-hourly. Only lowest doses required for nausea.

Contraindications: Parkinson's disease, coma. Use with caution in patients with severe cardiovascular problems; because of possible hypotension. Thyrotoxicosis (extrapyramidal problems more likely).

Common adverse effects: extrapyramidal symptoms, eg. akathisia, dyskinesia, akinesia, dystonias, Parkinsonism, sedation, neuroleptic malignant syndrome. Reduce dose in elderly patients.

Interactions: *increased adverse effects with* indomethacin (drowsiness), fluoxetine, metoclopramide (extrapyramidal effects), cimetidine; *action of haloperidol reduced by* rifampicin, carbamazepine. Use with lithium causes lethargy, fever, confusion and severe extrapyramidal symptoms.

hydromorphone

(4.7.2. Opioid analgesics)

PO.

Preparations: capsules (Palladone, Palladone SR).

Indications: opioid sensitive pain. Pain in the presence of renal impairment.

Action: strong stimulation of opioid *mu-receptors.*

Dose: dose titrated to individual patient. Four hourly (Palladone) or 12-hourly (Palladone SR).

Children:[2] oral starting doses (not previously on an opioid)- <50kg = 20microg./kg 4-6 hourly; >50kg = 3mg 3-4 hourly (halve these doses for parenteral administration).

Contraindications: no absolute contraindications in patients with advanced disease.

Common adverse effects: as for morphine.

Interactions: *adverse effects enhanced by* other CNS depressants and cimetidine; *reduces the action of* mexiletine; hypertension or hypotension may occur with MAOIs.

Comments: oral bioavailability about 60%. Approximately 7.5 times as potent as morphine by mouth,[24] although one study suggests the ratio may be closer to 4 : 1.[25] Appears not to have any active, renally excreted metabolites. Since it does not have the complex pharmacokinetics of methadone or transdermal fentanyl, it is the preferred alternative to morphine, but in the UK has no parenteral preparation.

hyoscine butylbromide

(1.2. Antispasmodics and other drugs altering gut)

IV, SC, IM.

Preparations: injection (Buscopan).

Indications: smooth muscle spasm (colic); bronchial secretions; inoperable bowel obstruction.

Action: antimuscarinic and antisecretory.

Dose: 20mg via the parenteral route repeated as required, or 30-180mg SC infusion per 24 hours.

Children: 25 microg./kg/hr infusion.

Contraindications: in long term use – closed angle glaucoma.

Common adverse effects: quaternary derivatives such as butylbromide do not readily cross the blood-brain barrier, so central effects are uncommon, but adverse effects similar to hyoscine hydrobromide can occur.

Interactions: *as for hyoscine hydrobromide.*

Comments: poor oral absorption (~ 10%).

---

hyoscine hydrobromide

(4.6 Drugs used in nausea and vertigo)

SL, SC, transdermal.

Preparations: tablets (Kwells, Joy Rides); transdermal (Scopoderm); injection (NP).

Indications: bronchial secretions at the end of life; inoperable bowel obstruction.

Action: antimuscarinic and antisecretory.

Dose: SC: 200 to 400 microg. 2-hourly as required, or 600-1200microg. SC infusion per 24 hours. Transdermal: each patch delivers approximately 150microg/24 hours over 3 days.

Children: PO: 5microg./kg 6-hourly. SC: 5 microg./kg. as single dose (or 1microg./kg/hr infusion). Transdermal: < 4 years = half patch (approx. 75 microg/24 hours); > 4 years = whole patch

Contraindications: in long-term use- closed angle glaucoma. No absolute contraindications for managing bronchial secretions in the last hours and days of life.

Common adverse effects: tachycardia, drowsiness, dry mouth, blurred vision, flushed face, amnesia; central stimulation may precede depression, urinary retention, may worsen existing cardiac insufficiency.

Interactions: *increased adverse effects with* antidepressants, other antimuscarinics, antihistamines, antipsychotics; *reduces the action of* ketoconazole.

Comments: well absorbed via the skin. More costly than hyoscine butylbromide.

---

ibuprofen

(10.1.1. Non-steroidal anti-inflammatory drugs)

PO, topical.

Preparations: tablets (NP, Apsifen, Arthrofen, Brufen, Brufen Retard, Ebufac, Isisfen, Ibular, Lidifen, Mortrin, Rimofen, plus 17 brands available direct to the public); capsules (Fenbid); solution (Brufen); topical (Ibugel, Ibuspray, Proflex).

Indications: pain due to inflammation; bone pain unresponsive to opioids whilst awaiting other treatments.

Action: reduction of prostaglandin synthesis.

Dose: 400-800mg 8-hourly.

Children:[2] <7kg: not recommended. > 7kg 5-10mg/kg 8-hourly.

Contraindications: as for diclofenac.

Common adverse effects: has the lowest risk of gastrointestinal adverse effects of all NSAID's. At initiation of therapy: epigastric pain, nausea, diarrhoea, headache, slight dizziness. GI ulceration with melaena and/or haematemesis are a risk, especially in ill patients. *NB: H_2 antagonists <u>do not</u> prevent gastric ulceration due to NSAIDs.* Any part of the bowel can be affected [53, 54] and the elderly may ulcerate without pain. [55] Renal damage can occur. [56] Toxicity persists even a year after exposure.[83]

Interactions: as for diclofenac.

Comments: useful topically for pain relief in skin ulcers. Short acting with the least risk of adverse effects.[51]

imipramine
(4.3.1. Tricyclic and other antidepressant drugs)

PO

Preparations: tablets (NP, Tofranil), solution (Tofranil).

Indications: depression, neuropathic pain.

Action: inhibition of presynaptic uptake of serotonin and noradrenaline.

Dose: neuropathic pain starting dose: 10-25mg at night; depression starting dose: 50mg at night. In both situations the dose can be titrated up to 150-200mg daily.

Children: [1] not recommended below 7 years; > 7 years = 1mg/kg.

Contraindications: recent myocardial infarction, heart block, porphyria, mania, severe liver impairment, history of epilepsy. Use with caution in patients with narrow angle glaucoma or urinary retention.

Common adverse effects: usual antimuscarinic effects: dry mouth, blurred vision, urinary retention, constipation, difficulty in visual accommodation, ileus, increased ocular pressure, sedation, tachycardia, postural hypotension, sweating, black tongue. Less sedating than amitriptyline.

Interactions: adverse effects of imipramine increased with nefopam, phenothiazines and cimetidine; do not give within 2 weeks treatment with MAOIs (monoamine oxidase inhibitors); *reduces the actions of* antiepileptics; *increases the actions* of baclofen.

Comments: some elderly patients will not tolerate starting doses above 10mg at night. Increase gradually as tolerated. Give as single night time dose to minimise impact of sedative and antimuscarinic effects. Converted to desipramine.

---

ketamine
(15.1.1. Intravenous anaesthetics)

SC, PO, IV

Preparations: injection (Ketalar).

Indications: neuropathic pain unresponsive to tricyclic antidepressants and/or anticonvulsants; severe pain unresponsive to opioids.[26 - 28] It may also have a role in movement-related bone pain and skin ulceration. Advice from a pain or palliative care specialist is recommended.

Actions: N-methyl D-aspartase (NMDA) receptor channel blocker.[29]

Dose: if starting dose required use 10mg SC or 30mg PO. Otherwise use SC infusion of 50-300mg per 24 hours or 100 - 400mg 6-hourly PO.

Children: extensive experience of its use in anaesthesia in children, but no information on analgesic doses although they are likely to be similar to adult analgesic doses.

Contraindications: hypertension, schizophrenia, acute psychosis.

Common adverse effects: dysphoria, hallucinations (especially on first dose since, in our experience, tolerance occurs rapidly within days), sedation, confusion, increased muscle tone. Neuropsychiatric effects may be reduced by the concurrent use of benzodiazepines. In higher doses, tachycardia and hypertension may occur.

Comments: ketamine can provide valuable analgesia in severe pain problems such as multiple bone metastases with skeletal instability, erosive lesions, and severe neuropathic pain. Test doses can be used but adverse effects may cause the patient to reject further doses. It seems well tolerated by SC infusion. The oral route can be used.[29 - 31] The analgesia from oral administration is greater than one would expect from the 20% bioavailability by this route,[29] and it seems reasonable to use a SC : PO ratio of 1:3 (ie. 1mg SC = 3mg PO) until definitive studies are done. The difference is due to an active metabolite, norketamine, which although is only a third as potent, when given orally it is produced in greater quantities than ketamine.

Obtaining ketamine in the UK: until an oral preparation becomes available in the UK, it is necessary to use the injection solution orally.[31] At the end of 1998 in the UK ketamine is available in hospitals, but at home it is necessary for the prescribing doctor to order ketamine on a named patient basis from the manufacturers, Parke-Davis (Tel 01703 620500).

ketoconazole

(5.2. Antifungal drugs)

PO.

Preparations: tablets (Nizoral); suspension (Nizoral).

Indications: 5 day treatment of oral or vaginal candida in advanced disease.

Action: antifungal.

Dose: 200 mg daily with food for 5 days; vaginal candidosis: 400mg daily for 5 days.

Children:[1] 3mg/kg once daily.

Contraindications: serious pre-existing liver disease. Do not use with cisapride.

Common adverse effects: nausea, vomiting, abdominal pain, headache, rashes. Asymptomatic elevation of liver enzymes and rarely, hepatitis (1 in 15,000 exposed individuals[32]). Irritation and dermatitis after topical application.

Interactions: action of ketoconazole reduced by antimuscarinics, antacids, cimetidine, rifampicin, phenytoin, ranitidine; *action of ketoconazole increased by* hydrochlorthiazide; *increases the action of* warfarin, sulphonylureas, phenytoin, midazolam; *reduces the action of* cisapride (risk of ventricular arryhthmias).

lactulose

(1.6.4. Osmotic laxatives)

PO.

Preparations: solution (NP, Duphalac, Osmolax, Laxose, Lactugel, Regulose); powder (Lactulose Dry, Duphalac Dry).

Indications: constipation in advanced disease.

Actions: osmotic laxative

Dose: 15 to 30 ml 12-hourly.

Children: widely used, but as in adults causes bloating and abdominal discomfort.

Contraindications: intestinal obstruction.

Common adverse effects: abdominal discomfort, flatulence and cramps.

Comments: full laxative effect may take 48 hours to develop.

levomepromazine (methotrimeprazine)

(4.2.1. Antipsychotic drugs)

PO, SC, IM, IV.

Preparations: tablets (Nozinan); injection (Nozinan).

Indications: low doses: nausea and vomiting; high doses: psychosis or severe agitation.

Action: $5HT_2$, D_2, α_1 and histamine receptor antagonist.[33]

Dose: antiemetic: 5-25 mg once at night. Psychosis or agitation: 25-100mg PO 8-hourly, or 50-300mg SC infusion over 24 hours.

Children:[1] 100microg./kg 12 hourly as antiemetic; for sedation use 250 microg./kg 4-8 hourly or 0.5-3 mg/kg/24 hours SC infusion.

Contraindications: epilepsy, parkinsonism, hypothyroidism, myaesthenia gravis. Use with caution in patients receiving anti-hypertensive agents (including spinal bupivacaine).

Common adverse effects: may cause severe hypotension, especially in elderly patients, although this is less likely with antiemetic doses. Extrapyramidal symptoms. Less SC skin reactions reported with isotonic parenteral formulation.

Interactions: fatality reported after concurrent use with pargyline (MAOI type A).

lofepramine
(4.3.1. Tricyclic and other antidepressant drugs)

PO.

Preparations: tablets (NP, Gamanil); solution (Lomont).
Indications: depression
Action: inhibition of serotonin and noradrenaline uptake.
Dose: 70 to 210 mg at night.
Children: not recommended.
Contraindications: use with caution in cases of severe cardiovascular, renal & hepatic disease.
Common adverse effects: lower incidence of anti-muscarinic side effects than amitriptyline and less cardiotoxic than other tricyclic antidepressants. For other effects see amitriptyline.
Interactions: increased side effects with nefopam; do not give within 2 weeks treatment with MAOIs (monoamine oxidase inhibitors); antagonism of anti-epileptics; increased antimuscarinic effects with phenothiazines; enhanced muscle relaxant effect of baclofen; plasma levels increased by cimetidine.

loperamide
(1.4.2. Antimotility drugs)

PO.

Preparations: capsules (NP, Diocaps, Imodium, LoperaGen, Norimode); solution (Imodium).
Indications: diarrhoea
Action: stimulates segmentation and mixing movements of bowel, with consequent reduction in bowel transit.
Dose: 4 mg stat; then 2 mg after each loose stool, up to 16mg daily.
Children:[1] 0-4 years = not recommended; 4-12 years = 1mg up to 6-hourly.
Contraindications: acute infective diarrhoea
Common adverse effects: abdominal pain & other GI disturbances including toxic megacolon, dry mouth, fatigue, skin rashes; occasional CNS depression.

lorazepam
(4.1.2. Anxiolytics, 4.8.1. Control of epilepsy & 15.1.4. Sedative and perioperative drugs)

PO, IM, IV

Preparations: tablets (NP, Ativan)
Indications: control of anxiety where sedation needs to be minimised.
Action: facilitation of GABA binding to GABA receptors.
Dose: 0.5 - 1mg 8-hourly
Children:[1] not recommended.
Contraindications: no absolute contraindications in advanced disease.
Common adverse effects: as diazepam but less sedating and shorter acting.
Interactions: see diazepam.
Comments: can be used sublingually.

medroxyprogesterone acetate
(6.4.1.2. Progestogens)

PO

Preparations: tablets (Provera).

Indications: treatment of breast cancer, alternative to corticosteroids in treating anorexia.

Action: in breast cancer, reduces the number of oestrogen receptors. In anorexia, has a glucocorticoid action.

Dose: 400mg daily

Children: no information.

Contraindications: severe arterial disease, hepatic impairment.

Common adverse effects: acne, urticaria, fluid retention, weight changes, GI disturbances.

Interactions: action reduced by aminoglutethemide.

Comments: has been shown to be effective in treating cachexia in cancer.[80]

methadone
(4.7.2. Opioid analgesics)

PO, SC

Preparations: tablets (Physeptone); solution (NP, Methodex); injection (NP, Physeptone).

Indications: opioid responsive pain in patients with renal failure or excessive adverse effects from morphine.

Action: strong stimulation of *mu* and *delta* opioid receptors. Non-specific NMDA antagonist.

Dose: dose <u>and</u> interval titrated to individual. The titration regimen is very different to morphine if accumulation is to be avoided.[34] If already on morphine start at 10% of morphine dose, but if not previously on a strong opioid start at no more than 5mg. Repeat this dose at onset of pain, but not less than 3 hours later. Allow the patient to adjust the dosing interval, but not the dose. Once this stabilises (usually at 4 - 7 days), give the total daily methadone dose 12-hourly. If necessary, this dose can be increased in 50% steps.

Children: methadone is used in paediatric palliative care,[2] but needs special care in its use. Dose recommendations are as follows: PO- <50kg = 200 microg./kg 12-24 hourly; >50kg = 10mg 8-12 hourly (halve doses for parenteral route). No information exists on titration of methadone in children, but is sensible to use the regimen suggested for adults since this avoids the risk of accumulation and is safer if there is a lack of cross-tolerance between strong opioids.

Contraindications: no absolute contraindications in advanced disease.

Common adverse effects: as for morphine, but may be less sedating.

Interactions: adverse effects enhanced by other CNS depressants and cimetidine; *action reduced* by rifampicin, phenytoin; *reduces the action of* mexiletine; hypertension or hypotension may occur with MAOIs; *increases the action of* zidovudine.

Comments: accumulates on regular dosing, probably due to extravascular binding acting as a sort of 'slow-release reservoir'. Analgesia and adverse effects are not affected by renal problems. It has weak NMDA antagonist activity which may explain why it is sometimes effective in morphine-insensitive pain.[35, 36]

methotrimeprazine
(4.2.1. Antipsychotic drugs)

See levomepromazine

metoclopramide
(4.6. Drugs used in nausea and vertigo)

PO, SC, IM, IV.

Preparations: tablets (NP, Gastroflux, Gastrobid Continus, Maxolon, Primperan, Parmid); capsules (Gastromax, Maxolon SR); solution (Maxolon, Primperan, Parmid); injection (NP, Maxalon).

Indications: reduced gastric or jejunal motility.

Action: $5HT_4$ agonist and D_2 antagonist speeding upper GI emptying.

Dose: 10-30mg mg PO 8-hourly, or 30-90mg SC infusion per 24 hours.

Children:[1] up to 10kg = 1mg 12-hourly; 10-14kg = 1mg 8-12 hourly; 15-19kg = 2mg 8-12 hourly; 20-29mg = 2.5mg 8-hourly; >30kg = 5mg 8-hourly. Daily dose should not exceed 500 microg/kg.

Contraindications: Increased risk of extra-pyramidal effects if given concurrently with drugs such as phenothiazines. Care with hepatic and renal impairment.

Common adverse effects: Extra-pyramidal effects; predominantly acute dystonias in younger patients & parkinsonian or tardive dyskinesia in elderly patients.

Interactions: increases the effects of paracetamol and opioid analgesics. Diminishes absorption of drugs absorbed from the stomach & enhances absorption from the small intestine.

metronidazole
(5.1.11. Metronidazole and tinidazole & 13.10.1. Antibacterial preparations)

PO, PR, topical, IV.

Preparations: tablets (NP, Flagyl, Metrolyl, Vaginyl); solution (NP, Flagyl S); suppositories (Flagyl, Metrolyl, Zadstat); topical (Anabact, Metrogel, Metrotop, Rozex); injection (NP, Flagyl, Metrolyl).

Indications: anaerobic infection producing systemic infection or malodour.

Action: active against anaerobic bacteria and protozoa.

Dose: 200-400mg PO 12-hourly to reduce smell from fungating tumours.

Children:[1] 7.5mg/kg 8-hourly

Contraindications: use with caution in patients with blood dyscrasias or active CNS infection. Reduce dose in severe liver disease & in the elderly. Alcohol: see comment below.

Common adverse effects: nausea, vomiting, unpleasant taste, furred tongue, GI disturbances.

Interactions: action increased by cimetidine; *action reduced* by phenobarbitone; *increases action of* warfarin and phenytoin.

Comments: In clinical practice, the interaction of metronidazole and alcohol is rare (no such reaction has been observed in 12 years at St. Oswald's Hospice). We advise our patients not to abstain from drinking alcohol whilst taking metronidazole. No well controlled trials comparing topical versus oral metronidazole for fungating tumours; topical preparation many times more expensive than oral therapy.

midazolam
(15.1.4. Sedative and analgesic peri-operative drugs)

SC, IM, IV, spinal.

Preparations: injection (Hypnovel).

Indications: titrated sedation.

Action: facilitation of GABA binding to GABA receptors.

Dose: 2.5-5mg SC as a single dose; 20mg to 200mg SC infusion per 24 hours. In IV sedation, the titration should be no faster than 1mg/min where previous requirements are unknown. It has the significant advantage of a short duration of action (most patients are fully awake within the hour). The aim is to titrate until the patient's eyes droop and speech becomes slurred, but to stop short of the patient losing consciousness

Children:[2] 20-100 microg./kg/hr infusion

Contraindications: No specific contraindications when used for sedation at the end of life.
Common adverse effects: as diazepam but much shorter acting.
Interactions: Erythromycin may inhibit metabolism of midazolam leading to enhanced therapeutic effect. Itraconazole, ketoconazole and possibly fluconazole increase the plasma concentration of midazolam. See diazepam.
Comments: reduce dose in elderly patients.

---

misoprostol
(1.3.4. Prostaglandin analogues)
PO

Preparations: tablets (Cytotec).
Indications: prevention of peptic ulceration by NSAIDs
Action: prostaglandin analogue.
Dose: 200 - 400 microg. 12-hourly.
Children:[1] not recommended.
Contraindications: pregnancy.
Common adverse effects: dose-related diarrhoea (which can be severe), abdominal pain, nausea, vomiting, flatulence, menorrhagia, dizziness.
Interactions: increased adverse effects with phenylbutazone.
Comments: useful in preventing NSAID-induced gastric ulceration. Do not take with food or antacids.

---

morphine
(4.7.2. Opioid analgesics)
PO, SC, IV, spinal.

Preparations: instant release tablets (Sevredol); controlled release tablets (MST Continus, Oramorph SR, Zomorph); controlled release capsules (MXL, Morcap SR); instant release solution (Oramorph); controlled release suspension (MST Continus granules); suppositories (NP); injection (NP).
Indications: opioid sensitive pain.
Action: stimulation of mu-opioid receptors.
Dose: dose range is 5-5000mg PO daily. Given 4-hourly, except for controlled release morphine which is given 12-hourly (eg. MST) or once daily (eg. MXL). Can be given by SC infusion, although diamorphine is usually used. Morphine epidural dose about 1/10 and intrathecal dose about 1/100 of IM/SC dose.
Children:[2] typical oral starting doses (not previously on an opioid). Instant release- <50kg = 160 microg./kg 4-6 hourly, >50kg = 7.5mg 3-4 hourly. Controlled release- <50kg = 500 microg./kg 12-hourly; >50kg = 25mg 8-12 hourly.
Contraindications: no absolute contraindications in advanced disease.
Common adverse effects: on initiating treatment some patients are troubled with drowsiness, nausea or confusion. With continuing treatment, constipation occurs in nearly all patients. At any time small pupils are common.
Interactions: adverse effects enhanced by other CNS depressants and cimetidine; *reduces the action of* mexiletine; hypertension or hypotension may occur with MAOIs.
Comments:. Use with caution in patients with impaired renal function. Once - daily preparations such as MXL are as effective as twice-daily preparations such as MST Continus. [84]

Morphine name in UK	Preparation	Typical length of action	Comments
MST Continus*	tablet	12 hours	
MST Continus granules*	mixed with water to form suspension	12 hours	* With controlled release preparations there is no need to use a loading dose of an instant release preparation
MXL*	capsule	24 hours	
morphine	suppositories	4 hours	
Morcap SR*	capsule	24 hours	
Oramorph	liquid	4 hours	
Oramorph SR*	tablet	12 hours	
Sevredol	tablet	4 hours	
Zomorph*	capsule	12 hours	

---

nabilone *(4.6. Drugs used in nausea and vertigo)*
PO.
Preparations: capsules (Nabilone).
Indications: persistent dyspnoea.
Action: acts by a combination of adrenergic and antimuscarinic bronchodilator effects on the airways, together with a central sedative effect.
Dose: 100-500 microg. 12-hourly.
***Children:*[1]** not recommended.
Contraindications: no absolute contra-indications.
Common adverse effects: drowsiness, vertigo, euphoria, dry mouth, ataxia, visual disturbance, dysphoria, hypotension, headache, nausea.
Interactions: alcohol, anxiolytics and hypnotics potentiate sedative effect.

---

nefopam *(4.7.1. Non-opioid analgesics)*
PO, IM.
Preparations: tablets (Acupan); injection (Acupan).
Indications: mild to moderate pain in patients intolerant of opioids.
Action: non-narcotic, non-opioid, centrally acting analgesic.
Dose: PO: start with 30mg 8-hourly. 60mg PO is approximately bioequivalent with 20mg IM.
***Children:*[1]** not recommended.
Contraindications: concurrent therapy with MAOIs; and in patients with seizures. Caution if used in those taking tricyclics or patients with urinary retention or glaucoma.
Common adverse effects: nausea, nervousness, urinary retention, dry mouth, light-headedness. Pain at sight of injection.
Interactions: *increased adverse effects* with antimuscarinics, MAOIs and tricyclic antidepressants.
Comments: centrally-acting agent whose precise mode of action remains unclear. Does not inhibit prostaglandin synthesis. It appears to be approximately 1/3 as potent as oral morphine. It is useful in the small number of patients who cannot tolerate even low dose morphine.

nitrous oxide

(15.1.2. Inhalational anaesthetics)

(mixed 1:1 with oxygen as Entonox)

Indications: control of brief pain (eg. during procedures).

Action: unknown.

Dose: inhaled under patient's control- inhalation should stop if any drowsiness occurs.

Common adverse effects: drowsiness.

Comments: This is a gas that produces analgesia directly (not by acting as an anaesthetic) and is therefore a nonopioid primary analgesic. It is useful for brief episodes of analgesia.

octreotide

(8.3.4. Hormone antagonists)

SC, IV.

Preparations: injection (Sandostatin).

Indications: entero-cutaneous fistulae; GI peptide-secreting tumours (eg. insulinoma, VIPoma); intractable diarrhoea.

Action: inhibitor of GI peptides and function (somatostatin analogue). Also inhibits insulin, growth hormone and glucagon.

Dose: 50mcg SC once or twice daily increasing to 200mcg 8-hourly according to response. Give between meals or at bedtime to reduce GI adverse effects.

Children: no information.

Contraindications: no absolute contraindications in advanced disease.

Common adverse effects: nausea, anorexia, vomiting, abdominal pain and bloating, diarrhoea, steatorrhoea. Hyperglycaemia may occur with long-term use.

Interactions: Reduces absorption of cyclosporin and cimetidine.

Comments: use with caution in diabetics; transient deterioration in glucose tolerance on initiation of therapy, may improve on long-term treatment. Clearance is halved in severe renal failure. Rotate sites to minimise pain on injection.

omeprazole

(1.3.5. Proton pump inhibitors)

PO.

Preparations: capsules (Losec).

Indications: second line treatment for peptic ulceration; Zollinger Ellison syndrome.

Action: supresses gastric acid secretion by inhibition of the H^+/K^+ ATPase enzyme system at the secretory surface of the parietal cells.

Dose: 20 to 40mg daily. Zollinger Ellison, 60mg initially then 20mg daily titrated to 60mg 12-hourly.

Children:[1] not recommended.

Contraindications: no absolute contra-indications.

Common adverse effects: headache, diarrhoea, rashes, pruritis, dizziness.

Interactions: *increase the action of* warfarin, phenytoin, diazepam; *reduces the action of* ketoconazole.

Comments: useful in preventing NSAID-induced gastric ulceration and with fewer adverse effects than misoprostol.

ondansetron

(4.6. Drugs used in nausea and vertigo)

PO, SC, IV.
Preparations: tablets (Zofran); syrup (Zofran); suppositories (Zofran); injection (Zofran).
Indications: chemotherapy induced emesis, may have a place in pruritis due to uraemia.[37]
Action: $5HT_3$ antagonist.
Dose: 8mg 12-hourly.
Children: 0-2 years = not recommended; >2 years = 100 microg./kg (maximum 4mg).
Contraindications: no absolute contra-indications in advanced disease.
Common adverse effects: constipation, headache, facial flushing, sensation of warmth over the stomach, hiccups.
Interactions: Efficacy may be enhanced by a single dose of dexamethasone 20mg (chemotherapy data).
Comments: maximum of 8mg daily in severe hepatic failure. If no benefit seen after 48 hours further improvement is unlikely. Expensive and of uncertain value in non-chemotherapy emesis related to advanced disease.

oxycodone

(4.7.2. Opioid analgesics)

PR, PO
Preparations: suppositories (special order from BCM Specials).
Indications: opioid-sensitive pain.
Action: stimulation of *mu*-opioid and κ-opioid receptors.
Dose: titrated to individual patient.
Children:[2] PO: <50kg = 100 microg./kg 4-hourly; >50kg = 5mg 4-hourly.
Contraindications: no absolute contra-indications in advanced disease.
Common adverse effects: as for morphine
Interactions: adverse effects enhanced by other CNS depressants and cimetidine; *reduces the action of* mexiletine; hypertension or hypotension may occur with MAOIs.
Comments: useful in suppository form 8-hourly as an alternative to subcutaneous infusions. Oral forms will soon be available.

pamidronate (disodium pamidronate)

(6.6.2. Bisphosphonates)

IV
Preparations: injection (Aredia Dry Powder)
Indications: hypercalcaemia of malignancy, painful bone metastases.
Action: inhibition of osteoclastic bone resorption.
Dose: 60-90mg in 500mls 0.9% saline as IV infusion over 2-4 hours.
Children: no information.
Contraindications: renal impairment, cardiac disease.
Common adverse effects: transient fever occasionally with high doses, transient hypocalcaemia.
Interactions: increased risk of hypocalcaemia with aminoglycosides.
Comments: compared with clodronate, pamidronate produces a more marked and prolonged improvement in calcium levels and pain levels.[38] Infusion times of 2-4 hours are as safe and effective as longer infusion times.[39] Doses of 60-90mg produce longer remissions,[40] but repeat infusions may be needed after 2-3 weeks.[41] Hypercalcaemia takes 2-3 days to respond, while bone pain can respond within 5 days.

papaveretum

Not recommended for use in advanced disease

This is a mixture of opium alkaloids. 10mg orally = 5mg of anhydrous morphine. Papaveretum injections have no place, and although aspirin and papaveretum tablets contain less than 0.2% morphine and are therefore exempt from Controlled Drug Regulations, there are no other advantages over simple morphine solution and a NSAID.

paracetamol

PO, PR.

Preparations: tablets (NP, Anadin Paracetamol, Feminax, Fenalgic, Medinal, Miradol, Paramin, Paldesic, Panadol, Paracets, Placidex, Resolve, Salzone); solution and dispersible tablets (NP plus wide range of preparations); suppositories (NP, Alvedon).

Indications: Useful in a variety of pains, including skeletal muscle pains and mild pains related to advanced disease. It has an antipyretic effect that will reduce temperature, making it useful in some infections where pyrexia is a problem. Although a weak analgesic, it can be useful even if the patient is already on a strong opioid.

Action: inhibits brain cyclo-oxygenase (COX).

Dose: 1g 4-hourly.

Children: 10-15mg/kg 4-6 hourly (5mg/kg if jaundiced).

Contraindications: no absolute contra-indications.

Common adverse effects: well tolerated. Doses of 1G 4-hourly do not produce adverse effects, and there are no reports of liver toxicity with doses of 4-6G daily in divided doses in cancer patients.[14] Occasional skin rash and other allergic manifestations. May cause fulminant hepatic failure and acute tubular necrosis in overdose.

Interactions: action increased by metoclopramide and domperidone; *action reduced* by antimuscarinic agents. Repeated doses may increase therapeutic response to warfarin (ie. increased INR).

pentazocine

Not recommended for use in advanced disease.

In patients with advanced disease this analgesic has a high incidence of causing dysphoria and hallucinations.

pethidine

Not recommended for use in advanced disease.

Its short duration of action of 2-3 hours[42] makes it impractical for use in the chronic pain of advanced disease. In addition, one of its metabolites, norpethidine, lowers the epileptic threshold.

phenazocine
PO, SL
Preparations: tablets (Narphen).
Indications: opioid-sensitive pain.
Action: strong opioid *mu-* receptor agonist.
Dose: titrated to individual.
Children:[1] not recommended.
Contraindications: no absolute contraindications in patients with advanced and progressing disease.
Common adverse effects: as for morphine.
Interactions: adverse effects enhanced by other CNS depressants and cimetidine; *reduces the action of* mexiletine; hypertension or hypotension may occur with MAOIs.
Comments: Can be given orally or sublingually every 8-hours. Although it is 5 times more potent than morphine, the single dose size available (5mg) limits titration to a narrow dose range.

phenobarbital (phenobarbitone)
PO, SC, IM, IV
Preparations: tablets (NP); solution (NP); injection (NP)
Indications: maintenance of seizure control requiring a non-oral route, terminal agitation.
Action: possibly through stabilising cell membranes and by enhancing GABA inhibition of synaptic transmission.
Dose: 50-200mg IV repeated after 6 hours if necessary (max. 600mg daily). Dilute 1 in 10 with water for IV administration.
Children: [1] 15mg/kg daily SC/IV single dose or 500 microg./kg/hour SC infusion.
Contraindications: no absolute contraindications in patients with advanced disease.
Common adverse effects: drowsiness, lethargy, mental depression, ataxia, skin reactions. In the elderly: paradoxical excitement, restlessness and confusion. In children: hyperkinesia.
Interactions: effect reduced by tricyclic antidepressants, mianserin and antipsychotics; *reduces the effects* of metronidazole and warfarin.
Comments: helpful in some patients whose agitation is persisting despite midazolam or methotrimeprazine.[81] Can be given as a continuous SC infusion.

propantheline
PO.
Preparations: tablets (Pro-Banthine).
Indications: urinary frequency; smooth muscle spasm.
Action: antimuscarinic.
Dose: 15mg to 30mg 8-hourly 1 hour before food & at bedtime.
Children:[1] not recommended.
Contraindications: reflux oesophagitis, pyloric obstruction.
Common adverse effects: as for hyoscine hydrobromide.
Interactions: as for hyoscine hydrobromide.
Comments: poorly absorbed with a high incidence of side effects. Use with caution in the elderly; (increase risk of glaucoma & urinary retention), patients with severe heart failure, arrhythmias hypertension and hyperthyroidism.

ranitidine

PO, IV.

Preparations: tablets (NP, Zantac); solution (Zantac); injection (Zantac).

Indications: peptic ulceration; steatorrhoea due to bile duct obstruction.

Action: H$_2$ receptor antagonist

Dose: gastric & duodenal ulceration- 300mg at night; NSAID-associated ulceration- 300mg 12-hourly.

Children: 2-4mg/kg 12-hourly (max. 300mg daily).

Contraindications: no absolute contraindications, but halve dose in severe renal impairment.

Common adverse effects: altered bowel habit, dizziness, rash, tiredness, confusion, liver damage, headache.

Interactions: does not inhibit cytochrome P450 mixed function oxygenase system. Ranitidine causes a rise in gastric pH which increases absorption of nifedipine.

Comments: H$_2$ antagonists <u>do not</u> protect against NSAID-induced gastric ulceration. Approximately three times more expensive than cimetidine, but has fewer drug interactions.

sodium valproate

PO, IV.

Preparations: tablets (NP, Epilim, Orlept); capsules (Convulese); solution (NP, Epilim); injection (Epilim).

Indications: neuropathic pain, control of seizures.

Action: possibly through stabilising cell membranes and by enhancing GABA inhibition of synaptic transmission.

Dose: 500mg at night, titrated if necessary to 1g at night.

Children[1]: 5-10mg/kg 12-hourly (maximum 35mg/kg daily).

Contraindications: active liver disease, family history of severe hepatic dysfunction, porhyria.

Common adverse effects: gastric irritation, nausea, tremor, increased appetite, transient hair loss, oedema, thrombocytopaemia.

Comments: useful in some neuropathic pain. [48]

spironolactone

PO.

Preparations: tablets (NP, Aldactone, Spiroctan, Spirospare, Spirolone, Laractone); capsules (Spiroctan); solution (NP: special order).

Indications: ascites (with frusemide).

Action: potassium sparing diuretic and aldosterone antagonist.

Dose: 100mg to 200mg once daily; in refractory cases up to 400mg daily in divided doses.

Children:[1] 1-1.5mg/kg 12-hourly

Contraindications: hyperkalaemia, anuria, acute renal insufficiency.

Common adverse effects: gastrointestinal disturbances, impotence, gynaecomastia, lethargy, headache, confusion, rashes, hyperkalaemia.

Interactions: increased risk of hyperkalaemia if given with NSAIDs or ACE inhibitors. Increase effect of antihypertensive agents.

sucralfate
(1.3. Ulcer healing drugs)

PO, topically.

Preparations: tablets (Antepsin); suspension (Antepsin).

Indications: external bleeding; upper GI bleeding; gastric ulcer.

Action: haemostatic agent; enhances gastric mucosal protection.

Dose: external- topically applied; upper GI- 2 grams as suspension every hour in acute bleed, then morning and night.

Children: as for adult doses.

Contraindications: no absolute contraindications.

Common adverse effects: well tolerated. Occasional constipation, diarrhoea , nausea, dry mouth, rash, pruritis, back pain, dizziness, insomnia & indigestion.

Interactions: do not give antacids for 30 minutes before or after sucralfate. *Reduces absorption* of ciprofloxacin, ofloxacin, tetracycline, warfarin, phenytoin, ketoconazole, throxine and theophylline & digoxin. Do not give these agents within 2 hours of sucralfate administration.

Comments: The suspension is more palatable.

---

tramadol
(4.7.2. Opioid analgesics)

PO

Preparations: tablets (Zydol, Zydol SR); capsules (Tramake, Zamadol, Zydol); injection (Zydol).

Indications: mild pain.

Action: weak *mu*-receptor stimulation; inhibition of 5HT and noradrenaline uptake.

Dose: 50-100mg 4-hourly.

Children:[1] not recommended.

Contraindications: see dihydrocodeine. Caution if history of epilepsy. Opioid effect may be potentiated in the presence of impaired renal function.[43]

Common adverse effects: orthostatic hypotension, hallucinations, confusion, nausea, constipation.

Interactions: use with caution with tricylcic and SSRI antidepressants as the seizure threshold may be lowered; *effect reduced* by carbamazepine, *effect increased* by quinine. *Increases the effect* of digoxin, warfarin.

Comments: opioid potency is similar to dihydrocodeine. It inhibits reuptake of 5HT and noradrenaline, and this may have a role in non-opioid sensitive pain.

---

tranexamic acid
(2.11. Antifibrinolytic drugs and haemostatics)

PO, IV, topical.

Preparations: tablets (Cyclokapron); solution (Cyclokapron); injection (Cyclokapron).

Indications: internal or external capillary bleeding.

Action: inhibition of plasmogen activation and of fibrinolysis.

Dose: up to 1.5G 6-hourly.

Children: no information.

Contraindications: thromboembolic disease, bleeding from the bladder. Reduce dose to twice daily when serum creatinine exceeds 120 micromol/L, once daily above 250 micromol/L.

Common adverse effects: dose-related nausea, vomiting & diarrhoea. Also causes headache, pruritis muscle pains and skin rash. Giddiness on rapid IV injection.

Comments: ethamsylate produces fewer adverse effects and should be tried first. Alternatively tranexamic acid can be used topically.

---

valproate

see sodium valproate

Analgesics

Definitions

(derived from Thompson JW)[44]

opiate = a product derived from the juice of the opium poppy (eg. codeine, morphine).

opioid = a directly acting compound specifically antagonised by naloxone.

opioid receptor = the specialised area of a cell that interacts with an opioid to produce a sequence of events that includes analgesia. There are four opioid receptors (μ-mu, ∂-delta, κ-kappa and ε-epsilon) of which only μ, κ, and ∂ produce analgesia.

opioid agonist = a compound that activates opioid receptors, initiating events that include analgesia.

opioid partial agonist/antagonist = a range of compounds that stimulate opioid receptors incompletely (eg. buprenorphine), or compete for morphine at one opioid receptor while stimulating other opioid receptors (eg. nalbuphine, pentazocine).

opioid antagonist = a compound that competes strongly with morphine at all three opioid receptors (eg. naloxone) with the effect of reversing the effects of morphine.

primary analgesic = a compound with intrinsic analgesic activity. Although nonsteroidal anti-inflammatory drugs produce much of their analgesia through an indirect (antiprostaglandin) mechanism, they do have weak intrinsic analgesic activity and are therefore primary analgesics.

secondary analgesic = a compound producing analgesia through a secondary mechanism. This group includes compounds with a clear action (eg. antibiotics, antispasmodics), and those whose action in relieving pain is unclear (eg. anticonvulsants, antidepressants).

Primary analgesics	Secondary analgesics
Nonopioids e.g.paracetamol (acetaminophen), nefopam	**Low dose antidepressants** e.g. amitriptyline, lofepramine
Weak opioid agonists e.g. codeine, dihydrocodeine, dextropropoxyphene	**Anticonvulsants** e.g. carbamazepine, sodium valproate
Strong opioid agonists e.g. morphine, diamorphine, hydromorphone	**Membrane stabilising drugs** e.g. flecainide, mexiletine
Opioid partial agonist/antagonists e.g. buprenorphine	**Adrenergic pathway modifiers** e.g. clonidine
Nonsteroidal anti-inflammatory drugs e.g. ibuprofen	**Corticosteroids** e.g. dexamethasone
NMDA antagonists e.g. ketamine	**Antispasmodics** e.g. hyoscine butylbromide
Nitrous oxide (1:1 with oxygen as Entonox)	**Antispastics** e.g. baclofen
	Antibiotics

Subcutaneous infusions

The usual indications for the use of a continuous subcutaneous infusion are the same as for parenteral administration. A variety of miniaturised pumps are available suitable for continuous subcutaneous infusion, but in the UK the commonest is the Graseby:

The Graseby syringe drivers: Battery-powered portable devices holds the medication reservoir in a disposable syringe (usually 10mL) and weighs about 175 grams, including the battery.

MS26 pump: calibrated in millimetres per 24 hours. Most common pump for continuous infusions.
MS16 pump: calibrated in millimetres per hour. Occasionally used for rapid or high volume infusions.

- To accurately deliver the 24 hour dose it is necessary to measure the length of the syringe barrel which contains the dose to be given. This allows for differing syringe sizes.
- Sufficient solution must be made to allow for priming of the connection line. Failure to do this will either a) result in the syringe becoming empty before the 24 hours have elapsed or b) the total dose delivered will be less than that prescribed. In this way errors in drug delivery may approach 10%. When assessing the capacity of lines it is important to consider the volume of the luer locks at either end. The Baxter Microvolume Extension Set has a total capacity of just under 0.5mL.
- A single activation of the booster button on the MS26 advances the syringe barrel 0.23mm. With a 20ml BD syringe in which the 24 hour dose is contained in 15mls, approximately 20 boosts would be required to deliver only 50% of the equivalent of a 4-hourly dose. Consequently this pump is not suitable for patient controlled analgesia and the patient's opioid requirements must be stabilised before continuous subcutaneous infusion is commenced.
- **Subcutaneous needles and catheters:** Subcutaneous plastic cannulae, eg. the Baxter Quik-Cath or the Becton Dickinson Insyte-W are often more comfortable for patients than inflexible metal butterfly needles. Plastic cannulae reduce local reactions and increase the time the cannulae can be left in place.[64] Where cannulae or butterfly needles are left in situ to give 'as required' bolus dose the line should be flushed with a little saline after the drug has been given to ensure complete delivery of the dose administered.

Drugs used by subcutaneous infusion

Diamorphine and hydromorphone are the opioids of choice for continuous subcutaneous infusion. This is simply on grounds of solubility. This is an important factor when considering that most patients with advanced disease have very little muscle mass or subcutaneous tissue and therefore large-volume painful injections must be avoided.

Diazepam (Roche), chlorpromazine and prochlorperazine are too irritant to be given by this route. Methotrimeprazine, haloperidol, hyoscine, metoclopramide and cyclizine are commonly used and important stability data is summarised below. Although subcutaneous administration of such drugs is common practice in palliative care, this use falls outside the Product Licence for these preparations.

Drug compatibility and stability

Not all drugs are suitable for subcutaneous administration because of limited aqueous solubility or extremes of pH.[85] It is sometimes necessary to give more than one drug by this method and whilst the clinical needs of the patient must remain paramount every effort should be made to ensure any drug combinations are both compatible and stable. The absence of cloudiness in the syringe does not guarantee either. The following simple precautions will minimise the risk of problems of incompatibility and instability:

- **do not mix more than two drugs in a syringe**
- **do not leave antiemetics in a syringe for more than 24 hours**
- **check with local hospital pharmacy before using unusual combinations**

1. **Diamorphine:** Allwood[58] tested diamorphine up to 20mg/mL using HPLC and found less than 5% degradation in plastic syringes at temperatures of between 18 and 22°C for about 18 days. Hanks et al[59] found a temperature and concentration dependent degradation of diamorphine with a corresponding increase in levels of 6-0-acetyl morphine and morphine. At 21°C diamorphine 250mg/ml showed a 7.9% degradation at 7 days and an 8.5% degradation at 14 days whilst the same concentration at 37°C showed a 35% degradation at 7 days and a 54% degradation at 14 days. However, the clinical consequences of degradation of diamorphine to 6-0-acetyl morphine are unlikely to be as serious as suggested by the degradation data. Although definitive clinical studies are still required it has been suggested that 6-0-acetyl morphine is approximately equipotent with diamorphine.[60] Sodium chloride may precipitate diamorphine from concentrated solutions at a pH above 5.5.[61]

2. **Cyclizine** lactate up to 10mg/mL is compatible with most concentrations of diamorphine HCl within the first 24 hours of mixing, but for storage up to 7 days, the cyclizine concentration needs to be below 6mg/ml.[58, 60, 63] There is also no significant degradation of cyclizine.[58] The addition of haloperidol to a diamorphine/cyclizine mixture does not affect compatibility or stability.[62]

3. **Haloperidol** has no significant effect on the stability of diamorphine. Concentrations of diamorphine up to 20mg/mL with haloperidol 0.75mg/mL show less than 5% degradation for up to 18 days in Water for Injection at room temperature. There is also no significant degradation of haloperidol over this period.[58] The addition of haloperidol to a diamorphine/cyclizine mixture does not affect compatibility of stability.[62]

4. **Metoclopramide** concentration up to 5mg/ml are compatible with diamorphine up to 150mg/mL with some discolouration of solution after 7 days. At this a 9% loss of opioid and an 8% loss of antiemetic occur. This degradation of metoclopramide is accompanied by a sharp drop in pH from 3.5 to 2.3.[63]

5. **Methotrimeprazine:** Diamorphine 1mg/mL is compatible with methotrimeprazine 0.25 mg/mL at room temperature and shows less then 5% degradation for up to 96 hours.

6. **Hyoscine:** Concentrations of diamorphine up to 150mg/mL are compatible with hyoscine butylbromide 20mg/mL and hyoscine hydrobromide 400mcg/mL with less then 7% degradation of diamorphine being evident after 7 days.[63]

7. **Local reactions** at the infusion site have been reported following subcutaneous infusions of a variety of drugs in patients with advanced disease. Cyclizine and levomepromazine (methotrimeprazine) both occasionally produce local reactions. Some drugs such as chlorpromazine are so irritant they should never be used subcutaneously. They may be related to the tonicity and concentration of solutions used as well as individual drugs, but the material of the cannulae is also a factor with plastic cannulae causing fewer reactions.[64]

Spinal analgesia

Indications

In recent years NMDA antagonists such as ketamine have been useful in situations where previously spinal analgesia was the only option, but the spinal route is still needed in some patients. Spinal analgesia has shown to be valuable in patients with complex pains that have not respond adequately to opioids, secondary analgesics, radiotherapy or other pain relief methods. [65-69] It has been of use in neuropathic pain,[65, 67] but also in chronic non-malignant pain,[69] and in children.[68]

Epidural or intrathecal?

The epidural route has been the traditional route and most experience is with this route for short term analgesia. There are a number of disadvantages of the epidural route, however:
- Insertion is technically difficult.
- A local anaesthetic bolus is often needed to test if the line is in position. This has its risks and, while it gives excellent analgesia, this is short-lived and pain returns before the correct dosing schedule is found over the next few days. In our experience, patients cope poorly with the rapidly changing pain levels.
- Because of the relatively large veins in the epidural space there is always a risk of intravenous administration of drug.
- There is constant risk that the catheter may erode into the intrathecal space which requires lower dosing schedules.
- If infection does involve the epidural space it can be difficult to eradicate and causes local scarring.

In contrast, the intrathecal route has none of these problems, and catheters have been left in place for up to 10 months,[72, 73] without local reactions to the catheter.[74] Comparisons between the two routes have shown the intrathecal route to be more suitable for home use.[75, 76] We now use the intrathecal route in all cases.

Which drugs?

Early experience was with opioids alone. Respiratory depression does not appear to be a problem when a patient has previously been on morphine for many weeks. Continuous infusions of morphine are as effective as intermittent bolus doses.[70] Opioids must be free of preservative and in this form both morphine and hydromorphone are suitable.[71] In the UK freeze dried diamorphine is also suitable and easily available. For patients with severe opioid-resistant pain, local anaesthetics alone will produce useful short term relief, but with the likelihood of tolerance developing within 1-2 weeks. A valuable alternative is to use a low dose strong opioid / bupivacaine mixture.[72, 73] This combination can be given to ambulant patients. Other drugs have been used, especially clonidine for neuropathic pain.[67] Drug mixture computability has a particular importance in intrathecal analgesia, but morphine and bupivacaine mixtures, with or without clonidine, are compatible and stable for up to 90 days.[77]

Problems with lines and drugs

Infection is a risk, but in 11 years we have had two treatable epidural infections, but no intrathecal infections, despite some patients having clear foci of concurrent infection. In contrast, one series of 92 cancer patients had 3 cases of meningitis following intrathecal analgesia,[66] although another series of 140 patients should no serious infections.[77] Dislodged catheters are the commonest problem, although this is greatly reduced when care is taken over the insertion, tunnelling and fixation of the catheter.[78] Another problem is CSF leakage but like others,[77] we have found this settles spontaneously, often within days. Portex filters can be left in place for up to 60 days and still retain their antibacterial function.[79]

Procedures

Spinal routes need practitioners skilled in the technique of catheter placement and a nursing team that understands spinal catheter care.

Opioid/bupivacaine dosing guidelines

- Most patients will need an opioid + bupivacaine in a mg: mg ratio of 1:10.
- Reduce systemic opioid by 30%.
- Use starting bupivacaine doses below.
- Increase spinal bupivacaine by 50% every 24 hours until pain relieved – stop short of sensory or motor loss (this may be difficult if nerve damage present).
- Continue to reduce systemic opioid in 30% steps as long as pain is controlled.

*   Bupivacaine on its own should only be used for analgesia needed less than 24 hours.
*   The intrathecal route should be used as the route of first choice.
*   Use continuous infusion to control pain - never bolus doses.
*   When using bupivacaine do not exceed the stated limits.
*   For simplicity, stay with 0.25% bupivacaine (i.e. do not change concentration).

Starting doses: 24 hour continuous infusion

Drug	Intrathecal	Epidural
Morphine alone <u>or</u> diamorphine alone	x 0.01 of 24 hour oral morphine dose = 24 hour spinal dose in mg	x 0.1 of 24 hour oral morphine dose = 24 hour spinal dose in mg
Fentanyl	x 0.5 of 24 hour oral morphine in mg = 24 hour spinal dose in <u>micrograms</u>	x 5 of 24 hour oral morphine in mg = 24 hour spinal dose in <u>micrograms</u>
Bupivacaine alone (0.25% = 2.5mg/ml)	Bupivacaine doses: Lumbar = 10mls / 24 hours Thoracic = 5mls / 24 hours **Do not exceed 2mls / hour**	Bupivacaine doses: Lumbar= 20mls / 24 hours Thoracic = 10mls / 24 hours **Do not exceed 5mls / hour**
Bupivacaine with morphine or diamorphine (0.25% = 2.5mg/ml)	Bupivacaine doses: Lumbar = 5mls / 24 hours Thoracic = 3mls / 24 hours **Do not exceed 2mls / hour**	Bupivacaine doses: Lumbar = 5mls / 24 hours Thoracic = 2.5mls / 24 hours **Do not exceed 5mls / hour**

Notes

1. A pain which is not responding to oral or parenteral opioid may still respond to the spinal route.

2. There is usually little benefit in titrating above the following 24 hour opioid doses:

morphine	30mg intrathecally,	300mg epidurally
diamorphine	30mg "	300mg "
fentanyl	1.5 microg. "	30 microg. "

3. For the intrathecal route, a morphine or diamorphine : bupivacaine ratio of 1:10 is usual. Patients with neuropathic pains may require proportionately more bupivacaine, but other patients will need proportionately more opioid.

4. Intrathecal bupivacaine should not exceed 2mls of 0.25% bupivacaine / hour (5mg / hour) since significant sensory or motor loss, or hypotension are likely. These effects may also be seen at doses below this dose rate. Most patients need between 5 - 15mls/24 hrs.

References

References are listed according the book sections:

Introduction (pp 1–10)

(Consequences of Advanced Disease; Managing Distress; Principles of Symptom Control; Eliciting the Current Problems)

1. McKeever M, Regnard C. Qualitative interviews. In, *Palliative Crisis Response Service (PCRS) Needs Assessment. Final Report: February 1997*. Newcastle: St. Oswald's Hospice. 1997.

2. Addington–Hall J, McCarthy M. Dying from cancer: results of a national population based investigation. *Palliative Medicine* 1995; **9**: 295–305.

3. Breitbart W. Pain in AIDS. In, Eds Jensen TS, Turner JA, Wiesenfeld–Hallin Z. *Pain*. Proceedings of the 8th World Congress on Pain. Progress in Pain Research and Management Vol 8. Seattle: IASP Press, 1997 pp 63–100

4. Larve F, Fontaine A, Colleau SM. Underestimation and undertreatment of pain in HIV disease: multicentre study. *British Medical Journal* 1997; **314**: 23–28.

5. Saunders CM. In, *The Management of Terminal Illness*. London: Hospital Medicine Publications, 1967.

6. Heron J. In, *Catharsis in Human Development*. London: British Postgraduate Medical Federation (University of London), 1977.

7. Liossi C, Mystakidou K. Heron's theory of human needs in palliative care. *European Journal of Palliative Care*, 1997; **4**: 32–35.

8. Gamlin R, Leyland M, Regnard C. Unit 3: Meeting the Psychological Needs of Patients. In, *CLIP Open Learning Series* Manchester: Hochland and Hochland 1998.

9. Sims S. The significance of touch in palliative care. *Palliative Medicine* 1988; **2**: 58–61.

10. Spiegel D. The use of hypnosis in controlling cancer pain. *CA* 1985; **35**: 221–231.

11. Hilgard ER and Hilgard JR. *Hypnosis in the Relief of Pain*. California: William Kaufman Inc 1975.

12. Connell C. Art therapy as part of a palliative care programme. *Palliative Medicine* 1992; **6**: 18–25.

13. Mandel SE. Music therapy in the hospice: 'Muscialive'. *Palliative Medicine* 1992; **5**: 155–160.

14. Kearney M. In, *Mortally Wounded: Stories of soul pain, death and healing*. Dublin: Mercier, 1996.

15. Stedeford A. A safe place to suffer. *Palliative Medicine* 1987; **1**: 73–74.

16. Twycross RG, Harcourt J, Bergl S. A survey of pain in patients with advanced cancer. *Journal of Pain and Symptom Management* 1996; **12**: 273–282.

17. Desbiens NA, Mueller–Rizner N, Commors AF, Wenger NS. The relationship of nausea and dyspnoea to pain in seriously ill patients. *Pain* 1997; **71**: 149–156.

18. Maguire P, Faulkner A, Regnard C. Eliciting the current problems. In, *Flow Diagrams in Advanced Cancer and Other Diseases* . London: Edward Arnold, 1995. pp 1–4.

19. Faulkner A, Booth K. Helping cancer patients disclose their concerns. *European Journal of Cancer* 1996; **32a**: 78–81.

20. Faulkner A, Maguire P, Regnard C. Breaking bad news. In, *Flow Diagrams in Advanced Cancer and other Diseases*. London: Edward Arnold, 1995, pp 86–91.

21. Vachon MLS. The emotional problems of the patient. In, Doyle D, Hanks GWC and MacDonald N eds. *The Oxford Textbook of Palliative Medicine, 2nd edition*. Oxford: Oxford Medical Publications, 1997 pp 883–907.
22. Faulkner A, Regnard C. Handling difficult questions. In, *Flow Diagrams in Advanced Cancer and other Diseases*. London: Edward Arnold, 1995, pp 92–95.
23. Buckman R. Communication in palliative care: a practical guide. In, Doyle D, Hanks GWC and MacDonald N eds. *The Oxford Textbook of Palliative Medicine, 2nd edition*. Oxford: Oxford Medical Publications, 1997 pp141–156.

Pain (pp 11–22)

1. McKeever M, Regnard C. Qualitative interviews. In, *Palliative Crisis Response Service (PCRS) Needs Assessment. Final Report: February 1997*. Newcastle: St. Oswald's Hospice. 1997.
2. Twycross RG. Pain and suffering. In, *Pain Relief in Advanced Cancer*. Edinburgh: Churchill Livingstone, 1995.
3. Kan MK. Palliation of bone pain in patients with metastatic cancer using strontium–89 (Metastron). *Cancer Nursing* 1995; **18**: 286–291.
4. Thompson JW, Regnard C. Pain. In, *Flow Diagrams in Advanced Cancer and Other Diseases* . London: Edward Arnold, 1995. pp 5–10.
5. Ernst DS, Brasher P, Hagen N *et al* A randomized, controlled trial of intravenous clodronate in patients with metastatic bone disease and pain. *Journal of Pain and Symptom Management* 1997; **13**: 319–326.
6. Ernst DS, MacDonald RN, Paterson HG *et al*. A double–blind, crossover trial of intravenous clodronate in metastatic bone pain. *Journal of Pain and Symptom Management* 1992; **7**: 4–11.
7. Hortobagyi GN, Theriault RL, Porter L *et al* Efficacy of pamidronate in reducing skeletal complications in patients with breast cancer and lytic bone metastases. *New England Journal of Medicine* 1996; **335**: 1785–1791.
8. Berenson JR, Lichtenstein A, Porter L *et al* Efficacy of pamidronate in reducing skeletal events in patients with advanced multiple myeloma. *New England Journal of Medicine* 1996; **334**: 488–493.
9. Travell, Simons. Myofascial pain. *In*, Wall PD and Melzack R, eds. *Textbook of Pain, 2nd edition*. Edinburgh: Churchill Livingstone, 1989
10. Back IN, Finlay I. Analgesic effect of topical opioids on painful skin ulcers. *Journal of Pain and Symptom Management* 1995; **10**: 493.
11. Krajnik M, Zylicz Z. Topical morphine for cutaneous cancer pain. *Palliative Medicine* 1997; **11**: 325–326.
12. Jepson BA. Relieving the pain of pressure sores. *Lancet* 1992; **339**: 504–504.
13. Portenoy RK. Cancer pain: pathophysiology and syndromes. *Lancet* 1992; **339**: 1026–1031.
14. Hanks GW and Justins DM. Cancer pain: management. *Lancet*, 1992; **339**: 1031–6.
15. World Health Organisation. Cancer Pain Relief. Geneva: World Health Organisation, 1986.
16. Portenoy RK, Thaler HT, Inturrisi CE *et al* The metabolite morphine–6–glucuronide contributes to the analgesia produced by morphine infusion in patients with pain and normal renal function. *Clinical Pharmacology and Therapeutics* 1992; **51**: 422–431.
17. Faura CC, Moore A, Horgan JF *et al*. Morphine and morphine–6–glucuronide plasma concentrations and effect in cancer pain. *Journal of Pain and Symptom Management*. 1996; **11**: 95–102.
18. Mazoit JX, Sardouk P, Zetlaoui P *et al*. Pharmacokinetics of unchanged morphine in normal and cirrhotic patients. *Anaesthesia and Analgesia*, 1987; **66**: 293–98.
19. Portenoy RK, Foley KM, Stulman J *et al*. Plasma morphine and morphine–6–glucuronide during chronic morphine therapy for cancer pain: plasma profiles, steady state concentrations and the consequences of renal failure. *Pain* 1991; **47**: 13–19.

20. Ashby M, Fleming, Wood M *et al* Plasma morphine and glucuronide (M3G and M6G) concentrations in hospice patients. *Journal of Pain and Symptom Management* 1997; **14**: 157–167.

21. Nilsson MI et al. Clinical pharmacokinetics of methadone. *Acta Anaesthesia Scandanavica Supplement* 1982; **74**: 66–69.

22. Gannon C. The use of methadone in the care of the dying. *European Journal of Palliative Care* 1997, **4**: 152–158.

23. Hoskin PJ, Poulain P, Hanks GW. Controlled–release morphine in cancer pain. Is a loading dose required when the formulation is changed? *Anaesthesia* 1989; **44**: 897–901.

24. Wilkinson TJ, Robinson BA, Begg EJ *et al* Pharmacokinetics and efficacy of rectal versus oral sustained release morphine in cancer patients. *Cancer Chemotherapy and Pharmacology* 1992; **31**: 251–254.

25. Campora E, Merlini L, Pace M *et al*. The incidence of narcotic–induced emesis**.** *Journal of Pain and Symptom Management.* 1991; **6**: 428–430.

26. White ID, Hoskin PJ, Hanks GW and Bliss JM. Morphine and dryness of the mouth**.** *British Medical Journal* 1989; **298**: 1222–1223.

27. Schug SA, Zech D, Grond S *et al*. A long term survey of morphine in cancer pain patients. *Journal of Pain and Symptom Management* 1992; **7**: 259–266.

28. Taub A. Opioid analgesics in the treatment of chronic intractable pain of non–neoplastic origin. In, *Narcotic Analgesics in Anaesthesiology* editors Kitahata LM and Collins JG. Baltimore: Williams and Wilkins, 1982. Pp 199–208.

29. Regnard CFB, Badger C. Opioids, sleep and the time of death. *Palliative Medicine* 1987; **1**: 107–110.

30. Vainio A, Ollila J, Matikainen E *et al* Driving ability in cancer patients receiving long–term morphine analgesia. *Lancet* 1995; **346**: 667–670.

31. Twycross R. Misunderstandings about morphine. In, *Pain Relief in Advanced Cancer* Edinburgh: Churchill Livingstone, 1994 pp333–347.

32. Walsh TD. Opiates and respiratory function in advanced cancer. *Recent Results in Cancer Research Vol 89*. Berlin: Springer–Verlag, 1984; 115–117.

33. Evans PJD. Narcotic addiction in patients with chronic pain. *Anaesthesia* 1981; **36**: 597–602.

34. Bruera E, Pereira J, Watanabe S *et al* Opioid rotation in patients with cancer pain. A comparison of dose ratios between methadone, hydromorphone, and morphine. *Cancer* 1996; **78**: 852–857.

35. Fallon M. Opioid rotation: does it have a role? *Palliative Medicine* 1997; **11**: 177–178.

Other physical symptoms (pp 23–62)

1. Desbiens NA, Mueller–Rizner N, Connors AF *et al* The relationship of nausea and dyspnoea to pain in seriously ill patients. *Pain* 1997; **71**: 149–156.

2. Donnelly, Walsh D. The symptoms of advanced cancer. *Seminars in oncology* 1995; **22**: 67–72.

3. Breitbart W. Pain in AIDS: a special case of neuropathic pain. In, *Abstracts: 8th World Congress on Pain.* Seattle: IASP Press, 1996 p329.

4. Hicks F, Corcoran G. Should hospices offer respite admission to patients with motor neurone disease? *Palliative Medicine* 1993; **7**: 145–150.

5. Winningham M, Nail L, Barton Burke M *et al* Fatigue and the cancer experience: the state of the knowledge. *Oncology Nurse Forum* 1994; **21**: 23–36.

6. Regnard C, Mannix K. Weakness and fatigue. In, *Flow Diagrams in Advanced Cancer and other Diseases.* London: Edward Arnold, 1995. pp64–67.

7. Richardson A, Ream E. The experience of fatigue and other symptoms in patients receiving chemotherapy. *European Journal of Cancer Care* 1996; **5**: 24–30.

8.   Gall H. The basis of fatigue: where does it come from? *European Journal of Cancer Care* 1996; **5**: 31–34.

9.   Glaus A, Crow R, Hammond S. A qualitative study to explore the concept of fatigue/tiredness in cancer patients and healthy individuals. *European Journal of Cancer Care* 1996; **5**: 8–23.

10. Richardson A. Fatigue in cancer patients: a review of the literature. *European Journal of Cancer Care* 1995; **4**: 20–32.

11. Elrington G. The Lambert–Eaton myaesthenic syndromes. *Palliative Medicine* 1992; **6**: 9–17.

12. Bain PG *et al*. Effects of intravenous immunoglobulin on muscle weakness and calcium channel autoantibodies in the Lambert–Eaton myaesthenic syndrome. *Neurology* 1996; **47**: 678–683.

13. Yarbro CH. Interventions for fatigue. *European Journal of Cancer Care* 1996; **5**: 35–38.

14. Irvine D, Vincent L, Craydon JE. The prevalence and correlates of fatigue in patients receiving treatment with chemotherapy and radiotherapy: a comparison with the fatigue experienced by healthy individuals. *Cancer Nursing* 1994; **17**: 367–378.

15. Hickok JT, Morrow GR, McDonald S, Bellg AJ. Frequency and correlates of fatigue in lung cancer patients receiving radiation therapy: implications for management. *Journal of Pain and Symptom Management* 1996; **11**: 370–377.

16. Greenberg DB, Sawicka J, Eisenthal S *et al* Fatigue syndromes due to localised radiation. *Journal of Pain and Symptom Management* 1992; **7**: 38–45.

17. Davies AN. The management of xerostomia: a review. *European Journal of Cancer Care* 1997; **6**: 209–214.

18. Clemons M, Regnard C, Appleton T. Alertness, cognition and morphine in patients with advanced cancer. *Cancer Treatment Reviews* 1996; **22**: 451–468.

19. Regnard C, Manx K. Reduced hydration and feeding. *Flow Diagrams in Advanced Cancer and other Diseases*. London: Edward Arnold, 1995. pp 25–28.

20. Joint working party of the National Council for Hospice and Palliative Care Services and the ethics committee of the Association for Palliative Medicine of Great Britain and Ireland. Artificial hydration (AH) for people who are terminally ill. *European Journal of Palliative Care* 1997; **4**: 124.

21. Dunphy K, Finlay I, Rathbone G, *et al* Rehydration in palliative and terminal care. *Palliative Medicine* 1995; **9**: 221–228.

22. Fainsinger RL, Bruera E. When to treat dehydration in a terminally patient? *Supportive Care in Cancer* 1997; **5**: 205–211.

23. Moody C. Taste acuity, appetite and zinc status in patients with terminal cancer: BSc thesis in Food and Human Nutrition. Newcastle: University of Newcastle upon Tyne (Department of Biological and Nutritional Sciences), 1997.

24. Willox JC, Corr J, Shaw J. *et al*. Prednisolone as an appetite stimulant in patients with cancer. *British Medical Journal* 1984; **288**: 27.

25. Downer S *et al*. A double blind placebo controlled trial of medroxyprogesterone acetate (MPA) in cancer cachexia. *British Journal of Cancer* 1993; **67**: 1102–1105.

26. Hull MA, Rawlings J, Murray J *et al*. Audit of outcome of long–term enteral nutrition by percutaneous endoscopic gastrostomy. *Lancet* 1993; **341**: 869–872.

27. Fainsinger RL, MacEachern T, Miller MJ *et al* The use of hypodermoclysis for rehydration in terminally ill cancer patients. *Journal of Pain and Symptom Management* 1994; **9**: 298–302.

28. Regnard CFB. Comparison of concentrations of hyaluronidase. *Journal of Pain and Symptom Management* 1996; **12**: 147.

29. Bruera E. Comparison of concentrations of hyaluronidase: author's response. *Journal of Pain and Symptom Management* 1996; **12**: 148.

30. Williams J, Copp G. Food presentation and the terminally ill. *Nursing Standard* 1990; **4**:29–32.

31. DeWys D. Changes in taste sensation and feeding behaviour in cancer patients: a review. *Journal of Human Nutrition* 1978; **32**: 447–453.

32. Regnard C, Fitton S. Mouth care. In, *Flow Diagrams in Advanced Cancer and other Diseases.* London: Edward Arnold, 1995. pp 22–24.

33. Sammon P, Page C, Shepherd G. Oral hygiene. *Nursing Times* 1987; **83**: 25–27.

34. Pritchard P, Walker VA. Mouth care. In, *Manual of Clinical Nursing Policies and Procedures: the Royal Marsden Hospital*, eds. Pritchard P, Walker VA. London: Harper and Row, 1984. pp273–284.

35. Zegarelli EV, Kutschner AH, Silvers HF *et al*. Triamcinalone acetanide in the treatment of acute and chronic lesions of the oral mucous membranes. *Oral Surgery* 1960; **13**: 170–175.

36. Merchant HW, Gangarosa LP, Glassman AB *et al*. Betamethasone–17– benzoate in the treatment of recurrent apthous ulcers. *Oral Surgery* 1978; **45**: 870–875.

37. Graykowski EA and Kingman A. Double blind trial of tetracycline in recurrent apthous ulceration. *Journal of Oral Pathology* 1978; **7**: 376–382.

38. Samaranayake LP, Yaacob HB. Classification of oral candidosis. In, Samaranayake LP and MacFarlane TW, eds, *Oral Candidosis* London: Wright (Butterworth), 1990. pp 124–132.

39. Finlay IG. Oral symptoms and candida in the terminally ill. *British Medical Journal* 1986; **292**: 592–593.

40. Burnie JP, Odds FC, Lee W *et al*. Outbreak of systemic Candida albicans in intensive care unit caused by cross– infection. *British Medical Journal* 1985; **290**: 746–748.

41. Boon JM, Lafeber HN, Mannetje AH *et al* Comparison of ketoconazole with nystatin in the treatment of newborns and infants with oral candidosis. *Mycosis* 1989; **32**: 312–315.

42. Regnard C. Single dose fluconazole versus five day ketoconazole in oral candidosis. *Palliative Medicine* 1994; **8:** 72–73.

43. Hay RJ. Ketoconazole: a reappraisal. *British Medical Journal* 1985; **290**: 260–261.

44. De Felici R, Johnson DG and Galgiani JM. Gynaecomastia with ketoconazole. *Antimicrobial Agents in Chemotherapy* 1981; **19**: 1073–1074.

45. Heiberg JK and Svejgaard E. Toxic hepatitis during ketoconazole treatment. *British Medical Journal* 1981; **283**: 825–826.

46. Lewis JH, Zimmerman HJ, Benson GD *et al*. Hepatic injury associated with ketoconazole therapy– analysis of 33 cases. *Gastroenterology* 1984; **86**: 503–513.

47. Van Drimmelen J, Rollins HF. Evaluation of a commonly used oral hygiene agent. *Nursing Research* 1969; **18**:327–332.

48. Sweeney MP, Bagg J, Baxter WP et al. Clinical trial of a mucin–containing oral spray for treatment of xerostamia in hospice patients. *Palliative Medicine* 1997; **11**: 225–232.

49. Wiley SB. Why glycerol and lemon juice? *American Journal of Nursing,* 1969; **69**: 342–344.

50. Solomon MA. Oral sucralfate suspension for mucositis. *New England Journal of Medicine* 1986; **315**: 459–60

51. Kim JH, Chu F, Lakshmi V, *et al*. A clinical study of benzydamine for the treatment of radiotherapy-induced mucositis of the oropharynx. *International Journal of Tissue Reactions* 1985; **7**: 215–218.

52. Godding EW. Therapeutic agents. *Management of Constipation* editors Avery Jones F and Godding EW. Oxford: Blackwell Scientific Publications 1972. pp 38–70.

53. Sykes NP. A clinical comparison of laxatives in a hospice. *Palliative Medicine* 1991; **5**: 307–14.

54. Regnard C. Constipation. In, *Flow Diagrams in Advanced Cancer and other Diseases.* London: Edward Arnold, 1995. pp 11–13.

55. Anonymous. Laxatives: replacing danthron. *Drug and Therapeutics Bulletin* 1988; **26**: 53–6.

56. Tapson VF, Hull RD. Management of venous thromboembolic disease: the impact of low molecular weight heparin. *Clinical Chest Medicine* 1995; **16**: 281–294.

57. Cantelino NL, Menzoian JO, Logerfo FW *et al* Clinical experience with vena caval filters in high risk patients. *Cancer* 1982; **50**: 341–344.

58. Launois S, Bizec JL *et al* Hiccup in adults: an overview. *European Respiratory Journal* 1993; **6**: 563–575

59. Guelaud C, Similowski *et al* Baclofen therapy for chronic hiccup. *European Respiratory Journal* 1995; **8**: 235–237.

60. Wilcock A, Twycross R. Midazolam for intractable hiccup. *Journal of Pain and Symptom Management* 1996; **12**: 59–61.

61. Ahmedzai S, Regnard C. Dyspnoea. In, *Flow Diagrams in Advanced Cancer and other Diseases.* London: Edward Arnold, 1995. pp 48–53.

62. Sutton PP, Gemmell HG, Innes *et al* Use of nebulised saline and nebulised terbutaline as an adjunct to chest physiotherapy. *Thorax* 1988; **43**: 57–60.

63. Gleeson C, Spencer D. Blood transfusion and its benefits in palliative care. *Palliative Medicine* 1995; **9**: 307–313.

64. Monti M *et al* Use of blood transfusions in terminally ill cancer patients admitted to a palliative care unit. *Journal of Pain and Symptom Management* 1996; **12**: 18–22.

65. Branthwaite MA. Mechanical ventilation at home. *British Medical Journal* 1989; **298**: 1409.

66. Branthwaite MA. Non–invasive and domiciliary ventilation: positive pressure techniques. *Thorax* 1991; **46**: 208–212.

67. Ahmedzai S, Carter R, Mills RJ, Moram F. Effects of nabilone on pulmonary function. *Proceedings of the Oxford Symposium on Cannabis.* Oxford: IRL Press, 1985: 371–78.

68. Filshie J, Penn K, Ashley S, Davis C. Acupuncture for the relief of cancer–related breathlessness. *Palliative Medicine* 1996; **10**: 145–150.

69. Corner J, Plant H, A'Hern R *et al* Non–pharmacological intervention for breathlessness in lung cancer. *Palliative Medicine* 1996; **10**: 299–305.

70. Bailey C. Nursing as therapy in the management of breathlessness in lung cancer. *European Journal of Cancer Care* 1995; **4**: 184–190.

71. Ahmedzai S. Palliation of respiratory symptoms. In, Doyle D, Hanks GWC and MacDonald N eds. *The Oxford Textbook of Palliative Medicine, 2nd edition.* Oxford: Oxford Medical Publications, 1997 p583–616.

72. Hanning CD, Alexander–Williams JM. Pulse oximetry: a practical review. *British Medical Journal* 1995; **311**: 367–370.

73. Tattersall MHN and Boyer MJ. Management of malignant pleural effusions. *Thorax* 1990; **45**: 81–2.

74. Little AG, Ferguson MK, Golimb HM *et al*. Pleuroperitoneal shunting for malignant pleural effusions. *Cancer* 1986; **58**: 2470–43.

75. Johnson MJ. Problems of anticoagulation within a palliative care setting: an audit of hospice inpatients taking warfarin. *Palliative Medicine* 1997; **11**: 306–312.

76. Walsh TD. Opiates and respiratory function in advanced cancer. *Recent Results in Cancer Research* 1984; **89**: 115–117.

77. Young IH, Daviskas E, Keena VA. Effect of low dose nebulised morphine on exercise endurance in patients with chronic lung disease. *Thorax* 1989; **44**: 387–90.

78. Farncombe M, Chater S, Gillin A. The use of nebulised opioids for breathlessness: a chart review. *Palliative Medicine* 1994; **8**: 306–312.

79. Rogers D, Barnes P. Opioid inhibition of neurally mediated mucus secretion in human bronchi. *Lancet* 1989; **335**: 930–932.

80. Davis C, Penn K, A'Herne R *et al*. Single dose randomised controlled trial of nebulised morphine in patients with cancer–related breathlessness. *Palliative Medicine* 1996; **10**: 64.

81. Zappetella G. Nebulised morphine in the palliation of dyspnoea. *Palliative Medicine* 1997; **11**: 267–275.

82. Davis CL. The use of nebulised drugs in palliating respiratory symptoms of malignant disease. *European Journal of Palliative Care* 1995; **2**: 9–15.

83. Davies CL. ABC of palliative care: Breathlessness, cough and other respiratory problems. *British Medical Journal* 1997; **315**: 931–934.

84. Twycross RG. Respiratory symptoms. In, *Symptom Management in Advanced Cancer* Oxford: Radcliffe Press, 1997 pp143–155.

85. Hanks GW. Antiemetics for terminal cancer patients. *Lancet* 1982; **i**: 1410.

86. Lichter I. Which antiemetic? *Journal of Palliative Care* 1993; **9**: 42–50.

87. Regnard C, Comiskey M. Nausea and vomiting. In, *Flow Diagrams in Advanced Cancer and other Diseases.* London: Edward Arnold, 1995. pp 14–18.

88. Peroutka SJ, Snyder SH. Antiemetics: Neurotransmitter receptor binding predicts therapeutic actions. *Lancet* 1982; **i**: 658–659.

89. Sanger GJ. The pharmacology of anti–emetic agents. In, *Emesis in Anti–cancer Therapy: Mechanisms and Treatment.* London: Chapman and Hall, 1993.179–210.

90. Isbister WH, Elder P, Symons L. Non–operative management of malignant intestinal obstruction. *Royal College of Surgeons of Edinburgh* 1990; **35**: 369–372.

91. Twycross R. The use of prokinetic drugs in palliative care. *European Journal of Palliative Care* 1995; **4**: 143–145.

92. Janssens J, Peeters TL, Vantrappen G *et al* Improvement of gastric emptying in diabetic gastroparesis by erythromycin: preliminary studies. *New England Journal of Medicine* 1990; **322**: 1028–1031.

93. Yeo CJ, Barry MK, Sauter PK *et al* Erythromycin accelerates gastric emptying after pancreaticoduodenectomy. *Annals of Surgery* 1993; **218**: 229–238.

94. Twycross RG, Barkby GD, Hallwood PM. The use of low dose levomepromazine (methotrimeprazine) in the management of nausea and vomiting. *Progress in Palliative Care* 1997; **5**: 49–53.

95. Currow DC, Coughlan M, Fardell B *et al* Use of ondansetron in palliative medicine. *Journal of Pain and Symptom Management* 1997; **13**: 302–307.

96. Ashby MA, Game PA, Devitt P, *et al*. Percutaneous gastrostomy as a venting procedure in palliative care. *Palliative Medicine* 1991; **5**:147–150.

97. Watson JP, Mannix KA, Matthewson K. Percutaneous endoscopic gastroenterostomy and jejunal extension for gastric stasis in pancreatic carcinoma. *Palliative Medicine* 1997; **11**: 407–410.

98. Dundee JW, McMillan C. Positive evidence for P6 acupuncture antiemesis, *Postgraduate Medical Journal* 1991; **67**: 417–422.

99. Regnard C. Dysphagia. In, ed. Bates TD, Contemporary Palliation of Difficult Symptoms. *Clinical Oncology: International Practice and Research,* 1988. London: Balliere Tindall.

100. Logemann JA. In, *Evaluation and treatment of swallowing disorders.*, 1983. San Diego: College Hill Press.

101. Mason R. Palliation of malignant dysphagia: an alternative to surgery. *Annals of the Royal College of Surgeons of England* 1996; **78**: 457–462.

102. Regnard C. Dysphagia. In, *Flow Diagrams in Advanced Cancer and other Diseases.* London: Edward Arnold, 1995. pp 19–21.

103. Trier JS and Bjorkman DJ. Esophageal, gastric and intestinal candidiasis. *American Journal of Medicine* 1984; **77**: 39–43.

104. Sheft DJ and Shrago G. Esophageal moniliasis, the spectrum of the disease. *Journal of the American Medical Association* 1970; **213**: 1859–1862.

105. Carter RL, Pittam MR, Tanner NSB. Pain and dysphagia in patients with squamous carcinomas of the head and neck: the role of perineural spread. *Journal of the Royal Society of Medicine* 1982; **75**: 598–606.

106. Leighton SEJ, Burton MJ, Lund WS *et al* Swallowing in motor neurone disease. *Journal of the Royal Society of Medicine* 1994; **87**: 801–805.

107. Brewster AE, Davidson SE, Makin WP *et al* Intraluminal brachytherapy using the high dose rate microselectron in the palliation of carcinoma of the oesophagus. *Clinical Oncology* 1995; **7**: 102–105.

108. Carter R, Smith JS, Anderson JR. Laser recanalization *versus* endoscopic intubation in the palliation of malignant dysphagia: a randomized prospective study. *British Journal of Surgery* 1992; **79**: 1167–1170.

109. Lewis–Jones CM, Sturgess R, Ellershaw JE. Laser therapy in the palliation of dysphagia in oesophageal malignancy. *Palliative Medicine* 1995; **9**: 327–330.

110. Tietjen TG, Pankaj JP, Kalloo AN. Management of malignant oesophageal stricture with oesophageal dilatation and oesophageal stents. *The Esophagus* 1994; **4**: 851–862.

111. Scott AG, Austin HE. Nasogastric feeding in the management of severe dysphagia in motor neurone disease. *Palliative Medicine* 1994; **8**: 45–49.

112. Park RHR, Allison MC, Lang J *et al* Randomised comparison of percutaneous gastrostomy and nasogastric tube feeding in patients with persisting neurological dysphagia. *British Medical Journal* 1992; **304**: 1406–1409.

113. Twycross R, Regnard C. Dysphagia, dyspepsia and hiccup. In, Doyle D, Hanks GWC and MacDonald N eds. *The Oxford Textbook of Palliative Medicine, 2nd edition.* Oxford: Oxford Medical Publications, 1997 pp499 –512.

114. Regnard C, Mannix K. Urinary problems. In, *Flow Diagrams in Advanced Cancer and other Diseases.* London: Edward Arnold, 1995. pp 39–43.

115. Anon. Urinary tract candidosis. *Lancet* 1988; **ii**: 1000–1002.

116. Flanagan PG *et al.* Evaluation of four screening tests for bacteriuria in elderly people. *Lancet* 1989, **i**: 1117–19.

117. Tremblay S, Labbé J. Crystal clear urine and infection. *Lancet* 1994; **343**: 479–480.

118. Clague JE, Horan MA. Urine culture in the elderly: author's reply. *Lancet* 1994; **344**: 1779–1780.

119. Anon. Urinary tract infection. *MeReC Bulletin* 1995; **6**: 29–32.

120. Bullock N, Whitaker RH. Massive bladder haemorrhage. *British Medical Journal* 1985; **291**: 1522–1523.

121. Bramble FJ, Morley R. Drug–induced cystitis: the need for vigilance. *British Journal of Urology* 1997; **79**: 3–7.

122. Rittig S, Knusden B, Sorensen S *et al.* Longterm double–blind crossover study of desmopressin intranasal spray in the management of nocturnal enuresis. In: Medow SR ed. *Desmopressin in nocturnal enuresis.* Sutton Coldfield: Horus Medical, 1989: 43–55.

123. Malone–Lee J, Fader M and Budden C. Urinary incontinence. In: Goodwill CJ, Chamberlain MA eds. *Rehabilitation of the physically disabled adult.* London: Croom Helm, 1988: 479–98.

124. Anonymous. Underused: intermittent self catheterisation. *Drug and Therapeutics Bulletin* 1991; **29**: 37–39.

125. Hunt G, Whitaker R, Oakeshott P. *The User's Guide to Intermittent Catheterisation.* London: Family Publications Ltd (in association with the British Medical Association), 1993.

126. Smith P, Bruera E. Management of malignant ureteral obstruction in the palliative care setting. *Journal of Pain and Symptom Management* 1995; **10**: 481–486.

127. Davies A, Wang S. Blood transfusions in patients with advanced cancer. *Journal of Pain and Symptom Management* 1997; **13**: 318.

128. Back IN, Finlay I. Analgesic effect of topical opioids on painful skin ulcers. *Journal of Pain and Symptom Management* 1995; **10**: 495.

129. Goode HF, Burns E, Walker BE. Vitamin C depletion and pressure sores in elderly patients with femoral neck fracture. *British Medical Journal* 1992; **305**: 925–927.

130. Dickerson JWT. Ascorbic acid, zinc and wound healing. *Journal of Wound Care* 1993; **2**: 350–353.

131. Bale S, Regnard C. Pressure sores. In, *Flow Diagrams in Advanced Cancer and other Diseases.* London: Edward Arnold, 1995, p54–56.

132. Birchall L. Making sense of pressure sore calculators. *Nursing Times* 1993; **89**: 34–37.

133. Hofman A, Geelkerken RH, Wille J *et al* Pressure sores and pressure–decreasing mattresses: controlled clinical trial. *The Lancet* 1994; **343**: 568–571.

134. Boardman M, Palmer K, Harding KG. Hue, saturation and intensity in the healing wound edge. *Journal of Wound Care* 1994; **3**: 314–319.

135. Lowthian P. Pressure sores: a search for definition. *Nursing Standard* 1994; **9**: 30 –32.

136. Reid J for the pressure sore classification consensus committee. Towards a consensus: classification of pressure sores. *Journal of Wound Care* 1994; **3**: 157–160.

137. Kiecolt–Glaser JK, Marucha PT, Malarkey WB *et al* Slowing of healing by psychological stress. *The Lancet* 1995; **346**: 1194–1196.

138. Bale S. A guide to wound debridement. *Journal of Wound Care* 1997; **6**: 179–182.

139. Glide S. Cleaning choices. *Nursing Times* 1997; **88**: 74–78.

140. Gilchrist B on behalf of the European Tissue Repair Society. Should iodine be recognised in wound management? *Journal of Wound Care* 1997; **6**: 148–150.

141. Miller M. The ideal healing environment. *Nursing Times* 1994; **90**: 62–68.

142. Turner TD. Semiocclusive and occlusive dressings. In, Ryan T. ed, An environment for healing: the role of occlusion. *Royal Society of Medicine Congress and Symposium Series* 1985; **88**: 5–14.

143. Bale S. Dressing leg ulcers. *Journal of District Nursing* 1987; **5**: 9–13.

144. Anonymous. Wound management products and elastic hosiery. In, *British National Formulary No 34 (September 1997).* London: British Medical Association and the Royal Pharmaceutical Society of Great Britain, 1997. p652.

145. Jepson BA. Relieving the pain of pressure sores. *Lancet* 1992; **339**: 503–4.

146. Saunders J, Regnard C. Malignant ulcers. In, *Flow Diagrams in Advanced Cancer and other Diseases.* London: Edward Arnold, 1995, p57–59.

147. Newman V, Allwood M and Oakes RA. The use of metronidazole gel to control the smell of malodorous lesions. *Palliative Medicine* 1989; **3**: 303–5.

148. Pringle WK. The management of patients with enterocutaneous fistulae. *Journal of Wound Care* 1995; **4**: 211–213.

149. Regnard C, Meehan S. The use of a silicone foam dressing in the management of malignant oral-cutaneous fistula. *British Journal of Clinical Practice* 1982; **36**: 243–245.

150. Regnard C, Ruckley R. Silastic foam dressing: an appraisal. *Annals of the Royal College of Surgeons of England* 1985; **67**: 271.

151. Grocott P. The latest on latex. *Nursing Times* 1992; **88**: 61–62.

152. Nubiola P, Badia JM, Martinez–Rodenas F, *et al.* Treatment of 27 postoperative enterocutaneous fistulas with the long half–life somatostatin analogue SMS 201–995. *Annals of Surgery* 1989; **210**: 56–8.

153. Aymard JP Lederlin P, Witz F *et al.* Cimetidine for pruritus in Hodgkin's disease. *British Medical Journal* 1980; **280**: 151–152.

154. Harrison AR, Littenberg G, Goldstein L *et al* Pruritis, cimetidine and polycythaemia. *New England Journal of Medicine* 1979; **300**: 433–434.

155. Raderer M, Müller C, Scheithauer W. Ondansetron for pruritis due to cholestasis. *New England Journal of Medicine* 1994; **330**: 1540.

156. Peer G, Kivity S, Agami O *et al* Randomised trial of maltrexone in uraemic patients. *Lancet* 1996; **348**: 1552–1554.

157. De Marchi S, Cecchin E, Villalta D *et al* . Relief of pruritus during drug erythropoeitin therapy in patients with uraemia. *New England Journal of Medicine* 1992; **326**: 969–74.

158. Twycross RG. Pruritus and pain in *en cuirass* breast cancer. *Lancet* 1981; **ii**: 696.

159. Regnard C. Use of low dose spinal thioridazine to control sweating in advanced cancer. *Palliative Medicine* 1996; **10:** 78–79.

160. Regnard C, Makin W. Bleeding. In, *Flow Diagrams in Advanced Cancer and other Diseases.* London: Edward Arnold, 1995, p44–47.

161. Hollander D, Tarnawski A. The protective and therapeutic mechanisms of sucralfate. *Scandinavian Journal of Gastroenterology* 1990; **25**(suppl 173): 1–5.

162. Regnard CFB. Control of bleeding in advanced cancer. *Lancet* 1991; **337**: 974.

163. Regnard CFB, Mannix K. Palliation of gastric carcinoma haemorrhage with sucralfate. *Palliative Medicine* 1990; **4**: 329–30.

164. McElligot E, Quigley C, Hanks GW. Tranaxamic acid and rectal bleeding. *Lancet* 1992; **337**: 431.

165. Dean A, Tuffin P. Fibrinolytic inhibitors for cancer–associated bleeding problems. *Journal of Pain and Symptom Management* 1997; **13**: 20–24.

166. Broadley KE, Kurowska A, Dick R *et al* The role of embolisation in palliative care. *Palliative Medicine* 1995; **9**: 331–335.

167. Lang EK, Deutsch JS, Goodman JR *et al* Transcatheter embolization of hypogastric branch arteries in the management of intractable bladder haemorrhage. *Journal of Urology* 1979; **121**: 30–36.

168. Appleton DS, Sibley GNA, Doyle PT. Internal iliac artery embolisation of bladder and prostate haemorrhage. *British Journal of Urology* 1988; **61**: 45–47.

169. Rankin EM, Rubens RD, Redy JF. Transcatheter embolisation to control severe bleeding in fungating breast cancer. *European Journal of Surgical Oncology* 1988; **14**: 27–32.

170. McQuillan RE, Grzybowska PH, Finlay IG *et al* Use of embolisation in palliative care. *Palliative Medicine* 1996; **10**: 169–172.

171. Cooper DL, Sandler AB, Wilson LD *et al*. Disseminated intravascular coagulation and excessive fibrinolysis in a patient with metastatic prostate cancer. *Cancer* 1992; **70**: 656–658.

172. Stubbing NJ, Bailey P, Poole M. Protocol for accurate assessment of ABPI in patients with leg ulcers. *Journal of Wound Care* 1997; **6**: 417–418.

173. Badger C, Regnard C. Oedema. In, *Flow Diagrams in Advanced Cancer and other Diseases.* London: Edward Arnold, 1995, p60–63.

174. Regnard C, Badger C, Mortimer P, Stephenson L *Lymphoedema: advice on treatment, 3rd edition.* Beaconsfield: Beaconsfield publishers, 1998.

175. Mortimer PS, Badger C, Hall JG. Lymphoedema. In, Doyle D, Hanks G and MacDonald N, eds. *Oxford Texbook of Palliative Medicine, 2nd edition.* Oxford: Oxford University Press, 1997 pp 657–665.

176. Földi E, Földi M, Clodius L. The lymphoedema chaos: a lancet. *Annals of Plastic Surgery* 1989; **22**: 505–515.

177. Regnard C. Bowel Obstruction. In, *Flow Diagrams in Advanced Cancer and other Diseases.* London: Edward Arnold, 1995, p29–31.

178. Glass RL and LeDuc RJ. Small intestinal obstruction from peritoneal carcinomatosis. *American Journal of Surgery* 1973; **125**: 316–317.

179. Bizer LS, Liebling RW, Delany HM et al. Small bowel obstruction. *Surgery* 1981; **89**: 407–413.

180. Baines M.The pathophysiology and management of malignant intestinal obstruction. In, Doyle D, Hanks G and MacDonald N, eds. *Oxford Textbook of Palliative Medicine 2nd edition.* Oxford: Oxford University Press, 1997 pp 526–534.

181. Tunca JC, Buchler DA, Mack EA *et al*. The management of ovarian–cancer–caused bowel obstruction. *Gynaecological Oncology.* 1981; **12**: 186–192.

182. Telerman A, Gerard B, Van den Heule *et al*. Gastrointestinal metastases from extra–abdominal tumours. *Endoscopy* 1985; **17**: 99–101.

183. Ketcham AS, Hoye RC, Pilch YH *et al*. Delayed intestinal obstruction following treatment for cancer. *Cancer* 1970; **25**: 406–410.

184. Khoo D *et al* Palliation of malignant intestinal obstruction using octreotide. *European Journal of Cancer* 1990; **30A**: 28–30.

185. Twycross RG. Alimentary Symptoms. In, *Symptom Management in Advanced Cancer*. Oxford: Radcliff Medical Press, 1997 p158–221

186. McIntyre N, Burroughs N. Cirrhosis, portal hypertension and ascites. In, Weatherall DJ, Ledingham JGG and Warrell DA eds. *Oxford Textbook of Medicine on CD–Rom* Oxford: Oxford University Press / Publishing BV, 1996. pp2085–2100. [CD–Rom version of third edition].

187. Pockros PJ, Reynolds TB. Rapid diuresis in patients with ascites from chronic liver disease: the importance of peripheral oedema. *Gastroenterology* 1986; **90**: 1827–33.

188. Regnard C, Mannix. Management of ascites. In, *Flow Diagrams in Advanced Cancer and other Diseases*. London: Edward Arnold, 1995, pp 36 –38.

189. Bain VG. Jaundice, ascites and hepatic encephalopathy. In, Doyle D, Hanks G and MacDonald N, eds. *Oxford Textbook of Palliative Medicine, 2nd edition*. Oxford: Oxford University Press, 1997 pp 557–571.

190. Parsons SL, Watson SA, Steele RJC. Malignant ascites. *British Journal of surgery* 1996; **83**: 6–14.

191. Runyon BA. Care of patients with ascites. *New England Journal of Medicine* 1994; **330**: 337–342.

192. Greenway B, Johnson PJ and Williams R. Control of malignant ascites with spironolactone. *British Journal of Surgery* 1982; **69**: 441–442.

193. Fogel MR et al. Diuresis in the ascitic patient: a randomised controlled trial of three regimens. *Journal of Clinical Gastroenterology* 1981; **3**(Suppl 1): 73–80.

194. Amiel SA, Blackburn AM and Rubens RD. Intravenous infusion of frusemide as treatment for ascites in malignant disease. *British Medical Journal* 1984; **288**: 1041.

195. Sharma S, Walsh D. Management of symptomatic ascites with diuretics: two case studies and a review of the literature. *Journal of Pain and Symptom Management* 1995; **10**: 237–242.

196. Rubinstein D, McInnes I and Dudley F. Morbidity and mortality after peritoneovenous shunt surgery for refractory ascites. *Gut* 1985; **26**: 1070–1073.

197. Tarin D, Price JE, Kettlewell MGW et al. Clinicopathological observations on metastases in man studied in patients with peritoneovenous shunts. *British Medical Journal* 1984; **288**: 749–751.

198. Regnard C, Mannix K. The control of diarrhoea. . In, *Flow Diagrams in Advanced Cancer and other Diseases*. London: Edward Arnold, 1995, p32–35.

199. Carpenter CCJ. Cholera. In, Weatherall DJ, Ledingham JGG and Warrell DA eds. *Oxford Textbook of Medicine on CD–Rom* Oxford: Oxford University Press/Publishing BV, 1996. pp576–580. [CD–Rom version of third edition].

200. Beddar SAM, Holden–Bennett L, McCormick AM. Development and evaluation or a protocol to manage faecal incontinence in the patient with cancer. *Journal of Palliative Care* 1997; **13**: 27–38.

201. Mennie AT et al. Treatment of radiation–induced gastrointestinal distress with acetylsalicylate. *Lancet* 1975; **ii**: 942–943.

202. Yeoh EK, Lui D and Lee NY. The mechanism of diarrhoea resulting from pelvic and abdominal radiotherapy; a prospective study using selenium–75 labelled conjugated bile acid and cobalt–58 labelled cyanocobalamin. *The British Journal of Radiology* 1984; **57**: 1131–1136.

203. Cello JP, Grendall JH, Basuk P *et al*. Effect of octreotide on refractory AIDS–associated diarrhea. *Annals of Internal Medicine*, 1991; **115**: 705–10.

204. Mercadante S. Diarrhoea in terminally ill patients: pathophysiology and treatment. *Journal of Pain and Symptom Management* 1995; **10**: 298–309.

205. Bell JI, Hockaday TDR. Diabetes mellitus. In, Weatherall DJ, Ledingham JGG and Warrell DA eds. *Oxford Textbook of Medicine on CD–Rom* Oxford: Oxford University Press/Publishing BV, 1996. pp1448–1504. [CD–Rom version of third edition].

206. Nelson K, Walsh D, Sheehan F. The cancer anorexia–cachexia syndrome. *Journal of Clinical Oncology* 1994; **12**: 213–225.

207. Bower M, Brazil L, Coombes RC. Endocrine and metabolic complications of advanced cancer. In, Doyle D, Hanks GWC and MacDonald N eds. *The Oxford Textbook of Palliative Medicine, 2nd edition.* Oxford: Oxford Medical Publications, 1997 p709–725.

208. Downer S *et al.* A double blind placebo controlled trial of medroxyprogesterone acetate (MPA) in cancer cachexia. *British Journal of Cancer* 1993; **67**: 1102–1105.

209. Ahmedzai S, Davis C. Nebulised drugs in palliative care. *Thorax* 1997; **52** (suppl 2): 575–577.

210. Jalan R, Hayes PC. Hepatic encephalopathy and ascites. *Lancet* 1997; **350**: 1309–1314.

Psychological symptoms (pp 63–72)

1. Simpson M. Therapeutic uses of truth. In, Wilkes E ed. *The Dying Patient.* Lancaster: MTP Press, 1982 pp256–262.

2. Stedeford A, Regnard C. Confusional states. In, *Flow Diagrams in Advanced Cancer and other Diseases.* London: Edward Arnold, 1995, p68–72.

3. Inouye SK, van Dyck CH, Alesi *et al.* Clarifying confusion: the confusion assessment method- a new method for detection of delerium. *Annals of Internal Medicine* 1990; **113**: 941–948.

4. Brittlebank A, Regnard C. Terror or depression? A case report. *Palliative Medicine* 1990; **4**: 317–319.

5. Stedeford A. Confusion. In, *Facing Death: patients, families and professionals, 2nd edition.* Oxford: Sobell Publications, 1994 pp149–163.

6. Maguire P, Faulkner A, Regnard C. The anxious person. In, *Flow Diagrams in Advanced Cancer and other Diseases.* London: Edward Arnold, 1995, p73–76.

7. Stockton M. Screening for depression and anxiety in the hospice inpatient population: validation study of three screening tools. In, *Fifth Congress of the European Association for Palliative Care (10–13 September 1997): Book of Abstracts* . London: EAPC/Marie Curie/APM. 1997 p 56.

8. Maguire P, Faulkner A, Regnard C. The withdrawn patient. In, *Flow Diagrams in Advanced Cancer and other Diseases.* London: Edward Arnold, 1995, pp 77–80.

9. Breibart W, Chochinov HV, Passik S. Psychiatric aspects of palliative care. In, Doyle D, Hanks GWC and MacDonald N eds. *The Oxford Textbook of Palliative Medicine, 2nd edition.* Oxford: Oxford Medical Publications, 1997 pp 933–954.

10. Urch CE, Field GB, Chamberlain JH. The drawback of HADS in assessment of depression in the inpatient and community palliative care setting. In, *Fifth Congress of the European Association for Palliative Care (10–13 September 1997): Book of Abstracts* . London: EAPC/Marie Curie/APM. 1997 p43.

11. Maguire P, Hopwood P, Tarrier N and Howell T. Treatment of depression in cancer patients. *Acta Psychiatrica Scandanavica* 1985; **72**: 81–84.

12. Zigmond AS, Snaith RP. The hospital anxiety and depression scale. *Acta Psychiatrica Scandanavica* 1983; **67**: 361–370.

13. Faulkner A, Maguire P, Regnard C. The angry person. In, *Flow Diagrams in Advanced Cancer and other Diseases.* London: Edward Arnold, 1995, pp 81–85.

14. Ramsay N. Referral to a liaison psychiatrist from a palliative care unit. *Palliative Medicine,* 1992. **6**: 54–60.

Emergencies (pp 73–82)

1. Rowell P. Intralesional methylprednisolone for rib metastases: an alternative to radiotherapy? *Palliative Medicine* 1988; **2**: 153–155.
2. Twycross RG. Pain and suffering. In, *Pain Relief in Advanced Cancer*. Edinburgh: Churchill Livingstone, 1995.
3. Striling C, Kurowska, Tookman A. Phenobarbitone in terminal restlessmess. In, *Fifth Congress of the European Association for Palliative Care (10–13 September 1997): Book of Abstracts* . London: EAPC/Marie Curie/APM. 1997 p 45.
4. Heath DA. Hypercalcaemia of malignancy. *Palliative Medicine* 1989; **3**: 1–11.
5. Bower M, Brazil L, Coombes RC. Endocrine and metabolic complications of advanced cancer. In, Doyle D, Hanks GWC and MacDonald N eds. *The Oxford Textbook of Palliative Medicine, 2nd edition*. Oxford: Oxford Medical Publications, 1997 p709–725.
6. Kovacs CS, MacDonald SM, Chik CL *et al*. Hypercalcaemia of malignancy in the palliative care patient: a treatment strategy. *Journal of Pain and Symptom Management* 1995; **10**: 224–232.
7. Iqbal SJ, Giles M, Ledger S *et al* Need for albumin adjustments of urgent total serum calcium. *Lancet* 1988; **ii**: 1477.
8. Gucalp R, Theirault R. Treatment of cancer–associated hypercalcaemia. *Archives of Internal Medicine* 1994; **154**: 1935–1944.
9. Wimalawansa SJ. Optimal frequency of administration of pamidronate in patients with hypercalcaemia of malignancy. *Clinical Endocrinology* 1994; **41**: 591–595.
10. Hoskin PJ. Radiotherapy in symptom management. In, Doyle D, Hanks GWC and MacDonald N eds.*The Oxford Textbook of Palliative Medicine, 2nd edition*. Oxford: Oxford Medical Publications, 1997 p275–6.
11. Jameson RM. Prolonged survival in paraplegia due to metastatic spinal tumours. *Lancet* 1974; **i**: 1209–1211.
12. Kramer JA. Spinal cord compression in malignancy. *Palliative Medicine* 1992; **6**: 202–211.
13. Bell JI, Hockaday TDR. Diabetes mellitus. In, Weatherall DJ, Ledingham JGG and Warrell DA eds. *Oxford Textbook of Medicine on CD–Rom* Oxford: Oxford University Press / Publishing BV, 1996. pp1448–1504. [CD–Rom version of third edition].
14. Poulson J. The management of diabetes in patients with advanced cancer. *Journal of Pain and Symptom Management* 1997; **13**: 339–346.
15. Bower M, Brazil L, Coombes RC. Endocrine and metabolic complications of advanced cancer. In, Doyle D, Hanks GWC and MacDonald N eds. *The Oxford Textbook of Palliative Medicine, 2nd edition*. Oxford: Oxford Medical Publications, 1997 p709–725.

Drug information (pp 83–120)

1. British National Formulary, number 34 (September, 1997). London: British Medical Association and Royal Pharmaceutical Society of Great Britain. 1997.
2. McGrath PA. Paediatric palliative care: pain control. In, Doyle D, Hanks GWC and MacDonald N eds. *The Oxford Textbook of Palliative Medicine, 2nd edition*. Oxford: Oxford Medical Publications, 1997 pp 1013–1031.
3. Goldman A. Life threatening illnesses and symptom control in children. In, Doyle D, Hanks GWC and MacDonald N eds. *The Oxford Textbook of Palliative Medicine, 2nd edition*. Oxford: Oxford Medical Publications, 1997 pp 1033–1043.
4. Melzack R, Mount BM. The Brompton mixture versus morphine solution given orally: effects on pain. *Canadian Medical Association Journal* 1979; **120**: 435–438.

5. Twycross RG, Gilhooley RA. Euphoriant elixirs (letter). *British Medical Journal* 1973; **2**: 552.

6. Twycross RG. Value of cocaine in opiate–containing elixirs (letter). *British Medical Journal* 1977; **2**: 1348.

7. Twycross R. The use of prokinetic drugs in palliative care. *European Journal of Palliative Care* 1995; **2**: 143–145.

8. Eisenach JC, DeKock M, Klimscha W. α_2–adrenergic agonists for regional anaesthesia. A review of clonidine (1984–1995). *Anaesthesiology* 1996; **85**: 655–674.

9. Hanks GW and Justins DM. Cancer pain: management. *Lancet*, 1992; **339**: 1031–6.

10. Caracini A, Martini C. Neurological problems. In, Doyle D, Hanks GWC and MacDonald N eds. *The Oxford Textbook of Palliative Medicine, 2nd edition.* Oxford: Oxford Medical Publications, 1997 pp 727–749.

11. Kirkham SR. The palliation of cerebral tumours with high dose dexamethasone: a review. *Palliative Medicine*, 1989; **2**: 27–33.

12. Jones TE, Morris RG, Saccoia NC, Thorne D. Dextromoramide pharmacokinetics following sublingual administration. *Palliative Medicine* 1996; **10**: 313–317.

13. Twycross RG. Choice of strong analgesic in terminal cancer: diamorphine or morphine? *Pain* 1977; **3**: 93–104.

14. Gorman DJ. Opioid analgesics in the management of pain in patients with cancer: an update. *Palliative Medicine* 1991; **5**: 277–194.

15. Gupta SK, Southam M, Gale R. System functionality and physiochemical model of fentanyl transdermal system. *Journal of Pain and Symptom Management* 1992; **7**(suppl): S17–S26.

16. Catterall RA. Problems of sweating and transdermal fentanyl. *Palliative Medicine* 1997; **??**: 169–170.

17. Ahmedzai F, Brooks D. On behalf of TTS – Fentanyl Comparitive Trial Group. Transdermal Fentanyl versus oral morphine in cancer pain: Preference: Efficacy and quality of life. **13:** 254–261.

18. Bruera E, Pereira J. Acute neuropsychiatric findings in a patient receiving fentanyl for cancer pain. *Pain* 1997; **69**: 199–201.

19. Lehmann KA, Zech D. Transdermal fentanyl: clinical pharmacology. *Journal of Pain and Symptom Management* 1992; **7**(suppl): S8–S16

20. Portenoy RK, Southam MA, Gupta SK *et al* Transdermal fentanyl for cancer pain. *Anaesthesiology* 1993; **78**: 36–43.

21. Gourlay GK, Mather LE. Postoperative pain management with TTS fentanyl: pharmacokinetics and pharmacodynamics. In: Lehmann KA, Zech D, eds. *Transdermal fentanyl*. Berlin: Springer, 1991: 1–7.

22. Simmonds MA, Richenbacher J. Transdermal fentanyl: long–term analgesic studies. *Journal of Pain and Symptom Management* 1992; **7**(suppl): S36–39.

23. Donner B *et al.* Direct conversion from oral morphine to transdermal fentanyl: a multicentre study in patients with cancer pain. *Pain* 1997; **64**: 527–534.

24. Twycross RG. Pain relief. In, *Symptom Management in Advanced Cancer* Oxford: Radcliffe Medical Press, 1997. pp36.

25. Lawlor P, Turner K, Hanson J, Bruera E. Dose ratio between morphine and hydromorphone in patients with cancer pain: a retrospective study. *Pain* 1997; **72**: 79–85

26. Mercadante S. Ketamine in cancer pain: an update. *Palliative Medicine* 1996; **10**: 225–230.

27. Fallon MT, Welsh J. The role of ketamine. *European Journal of Palliative Care* 1996; **3**: 143–146.

28. Laval G, Roisin D, Schaerer R. Intractable pain in the terminally ill. *European Journal of Palliative Medicine* 1997; **4**: 43–48.

29. Luczac J, Dickenson AH, Kotlinska–Lemieszek A. The role of ketamine, an NMDA receptor antagonist, in the management of pain. *Progress in Palliative Care* 1995; **3**: 127–134.

30. Grant IS, Nimmo WS, Clements JA. Pharmacokinetics and analgesics effects of IM and oral ketamine. *British Journal of Anaesthesia* 1981; **53**: 805–809.

31. Boradley KE, Kurowska A, Tookman A. Ketamine injection used orally. *Palliative Medicine* 1996; **10**: 247–250.

32. Lewis JH, Zimmerman HJ, Benson GD, Islak KG. Hepatic injury associated with ketoconazole therapy. *Gastroenterology* 1984; **86**: 503–513.

33. Twycross RG, Barkby D, Hallwood PM. The use of low dose levomepromazine (methotrimeprazine) in the management of nausea and vomiting. *Progress in Palliative Care* 1997; **5**: 49–53.

34. Gannon C. The use of methadone in the care of the dying. *European Journal of Palliative Care* 1997; **4**: 152–158.

35. Manfredi PL, Borsook D, Chandler SW, Payne R. Intravenous methadone for cancer pain unrelieved by morphine and hydromorphone: clinical observations. *Pain* 1997; **70**: 99–101.

36. Ripamonti C, Zeccz E, Bruera E. An update on the clinical use of methadone for cancer pain. *Pain* 1997; **70**: 109–115.

37. Raderer M, Müller C, Scheithauer W. Ondansetron for pruritis due to cholestasis. *New England Journal of Medicine* 1994; **330**: 1540.

38. Purohit OP, Radstone CR. A randomised double–blind comparison of intravenous pamidronate and clodronate in the treatment of hypercalcaemia of malignancy. *British Journal of Cancer* 1995; **72**: 1289–1293.

39. Dodwell DJ, Howell A. Infusion rate and pharmacokinetics if IV pamidronate in the treatment of tumour–induced hypercalcaemia. *Postgraduate Medical Journal* 1992; **62**: 434–439.

40. Nussbaum SR, Younger J, VandPol CJ et al. Single dose intravenous therapy with pamidronate for the treatment of hypercalcaemia of malignancy: comparison of 30–, 60–, and 90–mg dosages. *American Journal of Medicine* 1993; **95**: 297–304.

41. Wimalawansa SJ. Optimal frequency of administration of pamidronate in patients with hypercalcaemia of malignancy. *Clinical Endocrinology* 1994; **41**: 591–595.

42. Mather LE, Meffin PJ. Clinical pharmacokinetics of pethidine. *Clinical pharmacokinetics* 1978; **3**: 352–368.

43. Barnung SK, Treschow M, Borgbjerg FM. Respiratory depression following oral tramadol in a patient with impaired renal function. *Pain* 1997; **71**: 111–112.

44. Thompson JW. Clinical pharmacology of opioid agonists and partial agonists. *Royal Society of Medicine International Congress and Symposium Series*, 1990, **146**:17–38.

45. Portenoy RK. Issues in the management of neuropathic pain. In: Basbaum AI, Besson J–M, eds. In, *Towards a new pharmacotherapy of pain.* Chichester: Wiley, 1991: 393–414.

46. McQuay HJ, Tramèr M, Nye BA et al A systematic review of antidepressants in neuropathic pain. *Pain* 1996; **68**: 217–227.

47. Max MB, Lynch SA, Muir J et al Effects of desimipramine, amitriptyline and fluoxetine on pain in diabetic neuropathy. *New England Journal of Medicine* 1992; **47**: 1250–1256.

48. McQuay H, Carroll D, Jadad AR et al Anticonvulsant drugs in the management of pain: systematic review. *British Medical Journal* 1995; **311**: 1047–1052.

49. Guslandi M and Tittobello A. Steroid ulcers: a myth revisited. *British Medical Journal* 1992; **304**: 655–656.

50. Messer J, Reitman D, Sacks HS et al. Association of adrenocorticosteroid therapy and peptic-ulcer disease. *New England Journal of Medcine* 1983; **309:** 21–24.

51. Adams SS. Non–steroidal anti–inflammatory drugs, plasma half lives, and adverse reactions. *Lancet* 1987; **ii**: 1204–1205.

52. Anonymous. NSAIDs for renal and biliary colic: intramuscular diclofenac, *Drug and Therapeutics Bulletin* 1987; **25**: 85–86.

53. Editorial. NSAIDs and gut damage. *Lancet* 1989; **ii**: 600.

54. Bjarnason I, Prouse P, Smith T *et al.* Blood and protein loss via small–intestinal inflammation induced by non–steroidal anti–inflammatory drugs. *Lancet* 1987; **ii**: 711–713.

55. Skander MP and Ryan FP. Non–steroidal anti–inflammatory drugs and pain free peptic ulceration in the elderly. *British Medical Journal* 1988; **297**: 833–834.

56. Orme ML'E. Non–steroidal anti–inflammatory drugs and the kidney. *British Medical Journal* 1986; **292**:1622–23.

57. Editorial. Osteolytic metastases. *Lancet* 1976; **ii**: 1063–1064.

58. Allwood MC. The stability of diamorphine alone and in combination with antiemetics in plastic syringes. *Palliative Medicine* 1991; **5**:330–333.

59. Hanks GW et al. in *'Diamorphine. Its chemistry, pharmacology and clinical use'*. Ed D.Bruce Scott. London: Woodhead–Faulkner, 1988.

60. Wright CI, Barbour FA. The respiratory effects of morphine, codeine and related substances. *Journal of Pharmacology and Experimental Therapeutics* 1935, **54**: 25–33.

61. Martindale, ed JEF Reynolds, *The Extra Pharmacopeia*, 28th edition. London: The Pharmaceutical Press.

62. Grassby PF, Hutchings L. Drug combinations in syringe drivers: the compatibility of diamorphine with cyclizine and haloperidol. *Palliative Medicine* 1997; **11**: 217–224.

63. Regnard C, Pashley S, Westrope F. Antiemetic/diamorphine mixture compatibility in infusion pumps. *British Journal of Pharmaceutical Practice* 1986. **8**: 218–220.

64. Macmillan K, Bruera E, Kuehn N *et al.* A prospective comparison study between a butterfly needle and a Teflon cannula for subcutaneous narcotic administration. *Journal of Pain and Symptom Management* 1994; **9**: 82–84.

65. Hassenbusch SJ, Stanto–Hicks M, Conington EC *et al.* Long–term intraspinal infusions of opioids in the treatment of neuropathic pain. *Journal of Pain and Symptom Management* 1995; **7**: 529–543.

66. Devulder J, Ghys L, Dhondt W *et al.* Spinal analgesia in terminal care: risk verus benefit. *Journal of Pain and SymptomManagement* 1994; **9**: 75–81.

67. Eisencah JC, DuPen S, Dubois M. Epidural analgesia for intractable cancer pain. *Pain* 1995; **61**: 391–399.

68. Veyckemans F, Scholtes J–L, Ninane J. Cervical epidural analgesia for a cancer child at home. *Medical and Paediatric Oncology* 1994; **22**: 58–60.

69. Krames ES. Intraspinal opioid therapy for chronic nonmalignant pain: current practice and clinical guidelines. *Journal of Pain and Symptom Management* 1996; **11**: 333–352.

70. Gourlay GK, Plummer JL, Cherry DA *et al.* Comparison of intermittent bolus with continuous infusion of epidural morphine in the treatment of severe cancer pain. *Pain* 1991; **47**: 135–140.

71. de Castro J, Meynadier J and Zenz M. Drugs, In, *Regional Opioid Analgesia*; Dordrecht: Kluwer Academic, 1991.

72. Sjöberg M, Appelgren L, Einarsson S *et al.* Long term intrathecal morphine and bupivacaine in "refractory" cancer pain. I. Results from the first series of 52 patients. *Acta Anaesthesia Scandanavica* 1991; **35**: 30–43.

73. Sjöberg M, Nitescu P, Appelgren L *et al* Long–term intrathecal morphine and bupivacaine in patients with refractory cancer pain. *Anesthesiology* 1994; **80**: 284–297.

74. Sjöberg M, Karlsson PA, Nordborg C *et al* Neuropathological findings after long–term intrathecal infusion of morphine and bupivacaine for pain tretament in cancer patients. *Anesthesiology* 1992; **76**: 173–186.

75. Nitescu P, Appelgren L, Linder L–E *et al* Epidural versus intrathecal morphine–bupivacaine: assessment of consecutive tretaments in advanced cancer pain. *Journal of Pain and Symptom Management* 1990; **5**: 18–26.

76. Crul BJP and Delhass EM. Technical complications during longterm subarachnoid or epidural administration of morphine in terminally ill patients: a review of 140 cases. *Regional Anaesthesia* 1991; **16**: 209–213.

77. Wulf H, Gleim M, Mignat C. The stability of mixtures of morphine hydrochloride, bupivacaine hydrochloride and clonidine hydrochloride in portable pump reservoirs for the management of chronic pain syndromes. *Journal of Pain and Symptom Management* 1994; **9**: 308–311.

78. Nitescu P, Appelgren L, Hultman E *et al* Long–term, open catheterization of the spinal subarachnoid space for continuous infusion of narcotic and bupivacaine in patients with 'refractory' cancer pain. *The Clinical Journal of Pain* 1991; **7**: 143–161.

79. de Cicco M, Matovic M, Castellani GT *et al* Time–dependent efficacy of bacterial filters and infection risk in long–term epidural catheterization. *Anesthesiology* 1995; **82**: 765–771.

80. Downer S *et al.* A double blind placebo controlled trial of medroxyprogesterone acetate (MPA) in cancer cachexia. *British Journal of Cancer* 1993; **67**: 1102–1105.

81. Striling C, Kurowska, Tookman A. Phenobarbitone in terminal restlessmess. In, *Fifth Congress of the European Association for Palliative Care (10–13 September 1997): Book of Abstracts* . London: EAPC/Marie Curie/APM. 1997 p 45.

82. Zenz M, Donner B, Strumpf M. Withdrawal symptoms during therapy with housdual featanyl. *Journal of Pain and Symptom Management* 1994; **9**: 54–55.

83. MacDonald TM, Morant CV, Robinson GC *et al.* Association of upper gastrointestinal toxicity of non-steroidal anti-inflammatory drugs with continued exposure: Cohort study. *British Medical Journal* 1997; **315:** 1333–1337.

84. O'Brian TO, Mortimer PG, MacDonald CJ et al. Randomised crossover study comparing the ethicacy and tolerability of a novel once-daily morphine preparation (MXL capsules) with MST Continus tablets in cancer patients with severe pain. Palliative Medicine 1997; **11**: 475–482.

85. Twycross R, Wilcock A, Thorp S. *PCF1: Palliative Care Formulary.* Oxford: Radcliffe Medical Press, 1998.

Further reading

- Twycross R, Wilcock A, Thorp S. *PCF1: Palliative Care Formulary.* Oxford: Radcliffe Medical Press, 1998.

- Twycross RG. *Symptom Management in Advanced Cancer, 2nd edition.* Oxford: Radcliffe Medical Press, 1997.

- Doyle D, Hanks GWC and MacDonald N.*The Oxford Textbook of Palliative Medicine, 2nd edition.* Oxford: Oxford: Oxford Medical Publications, 1997.

- *British National Formulary* (produced twice yearly). London: British Medical Association and the Royal Pharmaceutical Society of Great Britain.

Index

A

acceptance 7
acetaminophen *see paracetamol*
acupuncture and acupressure
    dyspnoea 32
    nausea and vomiting 37
addiction to opioids 21
adrenocortical insufficiency 24
agitation 76
airway obstruction 32, 78
alertness 64, 65
ambivalence 7
amitriptyline 88
anaemia
    causing itching 48
    fatigue and weakness 25
    dyspnoea 33
anorexia 26, 27
frequency in cancer, AIDS and motor neurone disease 23
anger 70, 71
antiemetics 35, 36
antifungals 29
anxiety 66, 67
    anxiety state 67
    causing fatigue and weakness 25
    causing reduced hydration and feeding 26
    causing nausea and vomiting 36
    in confusion 64
apthous ulcers 28
area postrema 36, 55
ascites 56
aspiration 33, 38
autonomic insufficiency 59

B

baclofen 88
    hiccups 33
bad news 6
benzydamine
    oral spray 29
bisacodyl 89
bisphosphonates 77
bladder problems 39–43
bleeding 49–51
    urinary 39
bone
    fracture 12, 13
    metastases 14
    rib metastases 14

bowel obstruction 54, 55
breaking difficult news 6
breathlessness *see Dyspnoea*
Brompton cocktail 89
bronchial secretions at the end of life 32, 33
bupivacaine 89
    bladder pain 40
    paracentesis 57
buprenorphine 89

C

candidiasis
    oral 28, 29
    dysphagia 38
    itching 48
carbamazepine 90
carbenoxelone 29
carbocisteine 90
carcinoid 59
carmellose paste 29
catheter (urinary) 42, 43
cauda equinal lesion 79
cellulitis 48, 51, 53
chest infection 33, 34
children (starting doses for drugs) 83–86
cirrhosis 56,57
cisapride 35, 54, 90
clomipramine 67
clonidine 90
co-danthramer 30, 91
co-danthrusate 30, 91
codeine 92
cognitive therapy 46, 67, 70
coagulation disorders 49–51
colic 12, 75
    bladder 15, 40
    ureteric 15, 40
    bowel 54, 55
collusion
    by partner or relative 6
    by patient 7
concentration 64, 65
confusion *see Confusional states*
confusional states 64, 65
    caused by opioids 21
    causing incontinence 41
frequency in cancer, AIDS and motor neurone disease 23
constipation 30, 31
    as cause of bowel obstruction 54
    caused by opioids 21
frequency in cancer, AIDS and motor neurone disease 23
cough 33, 34
cord compression *see spinal cord compression*